Challenging Neuronormativity for Communal Justice

Armando M. Chilton

TABLE OF CONTENTS

ABSTRACT

This dissertation's primary goal is to trouble the ableism embedded in how written communication is taught and evaluated. Drawing on principles of disability justice, user experience (UX) design, and socially just writing assessment theory, I develop equity-oriented approaches to classroom grading, writing program directed self-placement, and theories of validity. I argue that for writing assessment ecologies to continue moving toward the goals of justice and equity, including intersectional anti-ableism, there must be commitments to crip community building, flexibility as access, radical trust, and participatory localization.

This dissertation thus examines how ableist norms, particularly those around neurodivergence (non-normative ways of thinking, behaving, and being), inform theories and practices across various writing assessment sites. In synthesizing multiple justice frameworks, I provide timely contributions (both theoretical and practical) to the aim of equity-oriented assessment methodologies. I focus on critiquing normative assumptions of how we value and support student writing so that we may improve students' learning conditions in our classrooms and beyond.

Chapter One

"Hope is the small hole cut into the honest machinery. The milk crate is still a milk crate, but with the right opening, a basketball can make its way through. If I am going to be afraid, I might as well do it honest. Arm in arm with everyone I love, adorned in blood and bruises, singing jokes on our way to a grave." –   *A Little Devil in America*

For the longest time, I didn't want to be a teacher. When I was in high school, I wanted to be a journalist, and when I was in college, I wanted to be an attorney. When I was eighteen, I took a summer job as a runner/receptionist for a legal firm dealing with bankruptcy, foreclosures, and evictions. The work was relatively simple: do the analog filing, reorganize the mess they called a filing system, "run" files to city hall and back, answer the phone, direct visitors to appropriate offices, fetch the attorney coffee, brew more coffee, and distribute/dispatch mail and packages. Some of my coworkers were kind, but many were impatient and refused to explain instructions more than once, and they often treated me as an outsider or a child (or both). Tasks assigned to me were dull and repetitive, so it wasn't long before I was bored and frustrated. My favorite part of the day was delivering and retrieving files from the waterfront municipal government office before the afternoon showers rolled in off the bay.

The combination of rude coworkers and the stress of mailing legal documents with intensely specific procedures was overwhelming, and I eventually started having panic attacks. Sometimes I had the foresight to walk out into the hot and humid Gulf Coast summer air and walk it off, but sometimes I didn't. My memories of being caught crouched and panicking are sun-bleached and blurry, framed by dark-red brick walls, the distant smell of dogwood tree blooms, and frowns of pity. When he learned about my "episode," the attorney who hired me called me into his office, asked me if I'd ever seen *Pulp Fiction*, and told me I needed to "calm the fuck down." He then reiterated that I was good at my job (even if the others were petty and cantankerous), that he had my back, and that I was *OK*. It's hard not to be resentful of the word when you hear it as frequently as I do: *You're OK. I'm OK. We're all OK. Stop crying—why are you still crying? Everything's A-OK. YOU—ARE—OK.*

Even if the coworkers had been pleasant and supportive, the gravity, urgency, and unending tensions of the work (of not accidentally ruining someone's life) were weights I felt I couldn't bear at the time. The stress bled like an ink stain through the entire office: the stifling air, coworkers sneaking cigarette breaks and drinking gallons of coffee, the unforgiving nature of the work. I didn't want anything to do with it. Looking back, of course, I can recognize a deeply ableist and inaccessible workplace. There was no patience for my ignorance or forgetfulness, no room for error. There were no accommodations for my anxiety or my undiagnosed ADHD; I had to "suck it up" and get all my work done. Sucking it up: a key ingredient in an ableist Slurpee.

I've never forgotten moments like this one with the attorney, moments of having to face the consequences of revealing I wasn't "OK," and that I have arguably never been "OK" by the standards of what Nick Walker (2021) (she/her pronouns) refers to as the pathology paradigm. In some contexts, the slippage of the mask invites harm; in others, it can feel like a weight lifted. Mia Mingus (2011; 2017) writes about the concept of access intimacy, which can be described as the feeling of that weight lifting or not existing at all. Mingus describes access intimacy as not just "helping" someone (2011) but as "interdependence in action" and a means of "queer[ing] access" (2017). As a vital part of transformative justice, access intimacy shifts access from the realm of logistics (the action of "helping" or "granting" access) to the realm of relationality, humanness, and community. According to the pathology paradigm, I didn't have any access needs in that law office: if I couldn't handle the pressure, it was my fault for being too emotional, too lazy, too stupid. Simply put, paradigms are ways of understanding the world around us— lenses to our realities—and their norms and beliefs are often so taken for granted they feel automatic, natural, and objectively true. In this project, the pathology paradigm is defined as the overarching set of beliefs and values around two assumptions. One, that there is one correct or proper way human minds function, and two, that if your ways of thinking and behaving don't adhere to those narrowly defined standards, you are sick, broken, abnormal, something to be fixed, and/or less than human. Essentially, the pathology paradigm convinces us to believe the following statement as objective truth: if your mind doesn't match the norm, "there is Something Wrong With You" (Walker, 2021, p. 18). How can I be "OK" when the pathology paradigm structures workplaces and educational institutions built on racist norms, competition, and inhumane production expectations? How are any of us "OK"?

Place & Positionality

I've always been chronically ill: there's no version of myself without asthma, without gastroenterology and dermatology issues, without lifelong fear of anaphylaxis, without POTS, without PMDD. One of my earliest memories is of the distinct metallic smell of the nebulizer and the humming buzz of the machine as I prepared my lungs for a full day of school. My body knows these histories; the body always remembers. But my anxiety and ADHD diagnoses came as an adult, and they put so much of my life (past and present) into perspective. So many things suddenly made sense. The lung-crushing fear of being *not OK* suddenly had context. In charting

the constellations of my neurodivergence, I became, as Ahmed (2017) says, a "retrospective

witness of [my] becoming" (p. 32). Disability communities offer the word "bodyminds" to resist

the false dichotomy: our minds and bodies are not discrete entities, nor are our logical and

emotional selves. We are whole beings, interconnected, and always in becoming.

In addition to neurodivergence and chronic illnesses, I'm a White[1] settler-colonizer who

currently lives and works on land seized from Indigenous Peoples and allocated to land-grant

universities in accordance with the Morrill Act, which was signed into law by President Lincoln

in 1862 (Ahtone, 2020; Lee & Ahtone, 2020; Lee et al., 2020). As a land-grant university, the

University of Arizona benefits from the possession of the traditional lands of the Tohono

O'odham Nation, whose predecessors include the Hohokam and the O'odham, as well as the

Pascua Yaqui Peoples. These communities have been continuously impacted by various

colonizers and land cessions.[2] It's important as scholars and teachers to understand the histories

of our institutions and the legacies of harm that sustain them (Vowel, 2016). I have also lived on

the ancestral lands of the Pensacola and Choctaw Peoples (Mobile, AL); the Pascagoula River

Tribe and Tunica-Biloxi Tribe (Bayou La Batre, AL); and the Muskogee Creek Indians and

Piqua Shawnee Tribe (Montevallo, AL; Birmingham, AL).[3] I share these histories and name

these peoples to acknowledge those harmed by centuries of colonialism but also to remember

---

[1] I capitalize White (as I will other races) in accordance with APA formatting and to underscore that White is not neutral or a standard race. Whiteness carries power and privilege that should be interrogated and denaturalized (for more information, see Nguyễn & Pendleton, 2020).

[2] Throughout the centuries, Tohono O'odham and Pascua Yaqui lands have been occupied by Spain, Mexico, the U.S., and the Confederacy. Government purchases for settlement expansion usurped the land, split the peoples between the U.S. and Mexico, and divided them into nine communities in Mexico, four U.S. federally recognized tribes (the Tohono O'odham Nation, the Gila River Indian Community, the Ak-Chin Indian Community, and the Salt River [Pima Maricopa] Indian community), and one non-federally recognized band, the Hia-C'ed O'odham (Tohono O'odham Nation, 2016).

[3] Like much of southeastern U.S., Alabama has extensive Indigenous histories. Many of its placenames are derived from that heritage ("List of Alabama placenames of Native American origin," 2023).

that sociocultural formations of disability were built (and are still concomitant with) legacies of colonialism, White supremacy, ethnocentrism, and xenophobia.

I live in proximity to a great deal of sociocultural privilege, especially as a White American citizen with English as their first language. As a White person in the United States, for example, I get to choose whether or not my research contributes to goals of racial justice and social/linguistic equity. Because I'm White, I can opt out of conversation about race; I can be "color blind" and ignore issues of race/ethnicity. I'm also a cisgender woman, which means I identify with the gender I was assigned at birth. While trans identities and gender fluidity are becoming more commonly accepted, there's still a great deal of violence (structural and interpersonal) inflicted upon those who stray from the traditional, normative boundaries of their assigned gender.[4] Women (and I use the word "women" as capaciously as possible) are still continually subjected to patriarchal violence and sexism in so many areas of their lives. Whether from sexual harassment at the gym, on public transportation, or in the workplace, to using a woman's ideas or her work without her permission or without citing her, sexism still shapes how I and many others move through the world. Being a woman also holds many social expectations of appearance, politeness, and performative happiness that limit or outright clash with some neurodivergent ways of being.

Disability and queerness are likewise interconnected. I identify as queer, particularly non-allonormative, and that's got a complicated history with disability justice.[5] People with disabilities are historically and problematically desexualized, *and*, also, many autistic and

---

[4] To learn more about the recent surge of anti-trans legislation in the United States, I suggest visiting the website www.translegislation.com, which tracks this information.

[5] Allonormativity is the set of norms and assumptions dictating compulsory sexual attraction. Amatonormativity is often used as the romantic attraction counterpart, though there's some debate about that (ace_arovolution, 2021a, 2021b). Here, I use "allonormative" to refer to norms governing both compulsory romantic attraction (alloromantic) and sexual attraction (allosexual). For more information, please see Smith College (n.d.) and Kassel (2021). I also use "aspec" or "A-spectrum" to indicate an identity relating to one or both of the asexual/aromantic spectrums.

disabled people identify as asexual and/or aromantic. Both statements are true and do coexist. M. Remi Yergeau (they/them pronouns) explains some of the tensions between disability and asexuality in *Authoring Autism*: "Those who embrace asexuality may be shamed or subject to reprimanding from disability rights activists, especially since disabled people have faced long histories of desexualization. … Even in queer circles, asexuality carries baggage" (2018, p. 190). Yergeau also discusses how asexuality, particularly demisexuality, invites examination of compulsory (allo)sexuality and other relationships to desire, not simply interrogating them but actively expanding (or exploding) them. Importantly, asexuality isn't celibacy, universality, or heteronormative—it is a queer "always becoming," one that challenges pervasive norms of attraction and longing (Yergeau, 2018, p. 189). For me and many others, weathering the ceaseless roar of allonormativity is as tedious as outdated gender expectations. By beginning the always-ongoing (and not untroubled) process of exploring and accepting my aspecness, my attunement to relationality has been radically refined and expanded: I find richness and wholeness in the contours of what's perceived as absence.

Identities, like minds, are kaleidoscopic. I'm a queer woman, a disabled teacher, and a first-generation graduate student all at once. These aren't pieces to break off and study; they're not LEGO® bricks. Because of the ways these converge, I experience various aspects of both privilege and marginalization, which have contextual and intersectional salience. What benefits me in some settings may be a source of limitations in others. It's important to note that "benefit" often means an absence of obstacles (meaning the benefits are unperceived, though still very real). This removal of obstacles is what so often signals privilege, and it's only in learning about what others face (and why/how) that we can begin collectively moving toward equity and justice. I've disclosed my positionality in this robust way because these confluences of identity directly impact my research and teaching, and because intersectionality is crucial to disability justice and other social justice work. As a foundational aspect of disability justice, intersectionality argues disability is always co-constructed alongside other social formations of race, gender, citizenship status, class, and sexuality. Importantly, intersectional frameworks dissect how these systems dynamically interconnect in ways that sustain ideologies and structures of domination and subordination (Crenshaw, 1991; Samuels, 2014). Leah Lakshmi Piepzna-Samarasinha (2018) (she/they pronouns) reminds us how "disability justice asserts that ableism helps make racism, christian supremacy, sexism, and queer- and transphobia possible, and that all those systems are locked up tight" (p. 22). To struggle with one is to struggle with all of them, which is why disability justice calls for cross-movement and cross-disability support and solidarity, and it's why disability justice calls for collective liberation: we leave no bodymind behind.

This project is not necessarily a happy one—happiness wasn't my aim. In fact, I come to this research curious, angry, exhausted, sad, *and* hopeful. They all coexist in a mélange of affective (dis)orientation. Ahmed (2017) writes about how happiness is socially constructed as many things: emotional labor, the expectation of a smile, avoidance of sadness, proximity to Whiteness, a tool of normative (re)direction. Taking unfamiliar or unexpected paths, deviating from norms, makes us subject to questioning about (un)happiness. Aspec people regularly hear such questions, often as warnings: You'll never be happy, or whole, or fully human without the love of a romantic partner! You can't be happy, or whole, or fully human without sex! Beware! Turn back now! These warnings are both value judgments and comfort zones. They are, as Ahmed (2017) so perfectly captures it, "just someone else's tired explanation" (p. 29). Ahmed also explains how heteronormativity is a "form of public comfort" (p. 123) because it creates and protects space for bodyminds who have already molded to that shape. Allonormativity and neuronormativity, I argue, function similarly. They are structural social comfort zones for those who inhabit them, which makes deviation and resistance uncomfortable. My panic attacks, for instance, make people uncomfortable: when they tell me I'm OK, what they're really saying is, "My comfort zone has been disturbed; your distress has made me not OK; I need you to be OK so that I can be OK." *Dry the tears. Suck it up. Breathe like a normal person. Let me back into my comfort zone.*

At the University of Montevallo (UM), my undergraduate alma mater, there's an annual event called the Life Raft Debate. Founded in 1998 by Dr. Michael Patton (University of Montevallo, 2018), the Life Raft Debate has a simple premise: there's been an apocalypse of some sort, and there's only room for one more person on the life raft to sustain the future all of humanity. Students gather in the gorgeous Palmer Hall auditorium to watch a handful of professors debate for their place on the raft, often through arguments about how their discipline(s), area(s) of expertise, and other skills/knowledges will be useful in establishing and maintaining a new civilization. There's also usually a Devil's Advocate, whose entire role is to convince the audience that *none* of the candidates are worthy of the final seat on the raft. Questions are raised about candidates' survivability, intelligence, and usefulness. Humor and quick wit are rewarded by laughter and votes. At the end of the debate, students vote for one of the professors (including the Devil's Advocate) to win. It's a fun event, even if professors take the earning of the coveted Life Raft Debate paddle very seriously, and students get to learn about the expertise of faculty from all over campus. I saw four of these debates in my time at UM, and I have a strong memory of Dr. Batkie, one of my English professors, giving an incredible recitation of several lines of *Beowulf* in fluent Old English (she won the paddle that year). In looking back, I realize how the Life Raft Debate is axiological, asking questions such as: What disciplines and types of knowledges do we value and why? What qualities of humanity do we value and why? When I'm examining various facets of equity and social justice, I often think about the Life Raft Debate—would an auditorium full of predominantly White, able-bodied undergraduates vote in favor of this thing being part of the future of humanity? Would most people resist the inclusion of disabled bodyminds on that life raft? It's a question many disability studies scholars and activists have been critically asking for some time: Who gets to survive and why? Who gets a future and why? Who's making those decisions and why?

Disability justice asserts that disabled bodyminds are just as valuable as temporarily abled ones, and it troubles the notion of a curative, eugenics-oriented, disability-free future.[6] As a framework and orientation, disability justice is the glue that holds the pieces of this project together. Born of the Disability Rights Movement, disability justice is both a continuation of that movement and a transformative justice framework: it seeks to reimagine, liberate, and empower through commitments to interdependence and collective care/action. Meaning we prioritize our commitments to people over institutions and to "critical connections over critical mass" (brown, 2017, p. 3). In this dissertation, I explore how these concepts can bolster the development of antiracist and justice-forward writing assessment ecologies. Building on Inoue's (2015) work, I define assessment ecologies as living, breathing, and always–in-becoming spaces, ones constituted by various stakeholders and participants (and their proximities to privilege and power). Ideally, justice-forward writing assessment ecologies support and make space for crip community building. Crip community building is a practice that prioritizes students' needs and knowledges, especially those of marginalized students, rather than privileging institutional expectations (currie & Hubrig, 2022; Kafai, 2021a, 2021b). In the classroom, crip community

---

[6] Patricia Berne, Mia Mingus, and Stacey Milbern (three incredible, disabled, queer women of color) gave us the transformative work of disability justice, now carried on by Sins Invalid and other networks of activists.

building compassionately asks teachers to prioritize relationships over efficiency, ethnocentric or racist notions of "excellence," control over students' behavior, productivity, or institutional alignment. "[Disability justice] means asserting a vision of liberation in which destroying ableism is part of social justice. It means the hotness, smarts, and value of our sick and disabled bodies. It means we are not left behind; we are beloved, kindred, needed" (Piepzna-Samarasinha, 2018, p. 22). It means making space on the life raft for folks who queer/resist/reimagine ableist standards of physical, neurological, behavioral, or emotional ability. In educational contexts, achieving these goals requires bridging the distance between theory and practice, between ideals and implementation. This dissertation seeks to do some of that bridge work.

Justice Frameworks

In my current professional context, I don't think I do disability justice. I certainly don't do it well or as well as I would like. Instead, I mostly do disability advocacy, with a lot of help from disability studies and its interdisciplinary connections to writing studies. Or perhaps it could be better described as anti-ableism: I do resistance work where and when I can, frequently asking instructors to think more carefully and compassionately about common practices in their classrooms and programs. Doing disability justice is a whole lot more than talking and reading and writing (though those components are necessary), and while justice and equity are often my conscious aims, there's plenty of room to err. Because disability isn't a monolith, there's no one right way to do disability justice, and it can look different depending on what's flaring, what's broken, what's aching that specific day. Piepzna-Samarasinha (2018) reiterates this point, adding, "Disability justice, when it's really happening, is too messy and wild to really fit into traditional movements and nonprofit industrial complex structures, because our bodies and minds are too wild to fit into those structures" (p. 124). Additionally, the phrase "disability justice" was and still is heavily co-opted by White disability scholars (including myself) without any critical interrogation of its histories or usage, and/or without citing the queer women of color involved in its inception (Sins Invalid, 2019), which is why I resist claiming this dissertation achieves those goals. But I would be lying if I said I didn't *dream* of disability justice, and it feels wrong to ignore the transformative framework developed by Berne, Mingus, and Milbern and their communities. To guide my research, there were many equity-oriented avenues I could have taken, and many frameworks could have been the backbone of this project. But the more widely I read, and the more I consciously encountered and resisted ableism in my daily professional work, I knew the work of Sins Invalid (2015, 2019) and activists/scholars like Piepzna-Samarasinha (2018) needed to be foregrounded in this project.

This dissertation is thus *inspired* by disability justice and makes many references to it, using its principles as guides and aims. This dissertation also begins with the assumption that theoretical and practical anti-ableist interventions are needed in our current academic landscape: I don't spend much time trying to convince any of my readers of the necessity of this work, though I do discuss the high-stakes nature of writing assessment and placement. With intention, I eschew the use of quantitative measurements to justify the need for disability activism or justice. I resist these rhetorics of fear, shock, and tragedy so that I can instead focus on stories, theories, histories, practices, and forward-looking pedagogies and initiatives. My paradigmatic approach to this project is informed by the principles of disability justice (Sins Invalid, 2015, 2019), technical and professional communication (TPC) design justice (Agboka, 2013; Costanza-Chock, 2020a), and the neurodiversity paradigm (Walker, 2021; Yergeau, 2018). These cross-

and interdisciplinary frameworks have some overlapping goals but offer diverse approaches to improving writing assessment for social justice, as I explore in each of the forthcoming chapters.

Additionally, a primary goal of this project is to examine sites of neuronormativity in writing assessment so that we may:

- Better understand the ways in which the pathology paradigm informs (and limits) traditional writing pedagogy and assessment; and

- Ideate and examine potential alternatives, ones that expand narrow notions of writing and thinking, and ones that honor the full humanity and valued complexity of all our students.

Neuronormativity is the package of socially constructed rules that substantiate and maintain the pathology paradigm—the set of ableist ideologies governing standards of thinking, learning, behaving, emoting, interacting socially, and being. For this project, I primarily use the term *neuronormativity* because it foregrounds the ways in which conventional conceptions of human minds are embedded in structures of ableist, White supremacist, cisheteropatriarchal, and imperial/colonial normativity and oppression. Additionally, as Nick Walker (2021) explains, "neurotypical" means living in and experiencing alignment with neuronormativity, not that someone is in possession of a "normal" brain—as I explain below, the neurodiversity paradigm doesn't believe there is a standard "normal" mind. I wanted a word for discussing norms of the pathology paradigm without associating all observations and analyses with neurotypicality, hence my use of "neuronormativity" and its variations. I also argue for replacing the pathology paradigm with the neurodiversity paradigm, as it offers more inclusive and more flexible ideologies. At its core, the neurodiversity paradigm believes there's no one correct way to exist, think, or behave. Walker (2021) summarizes it in three points:

- Neurodiversity—the diversity among minds—is a natural, healthy, and valuable form of human diversity.

- There is no "normal" or "right" style of human mind, any more than there is one "normal" or "right" ethnicity, gender, or culture.

- The social dynamics that manifest in regard to neurodiversity are similar to the social dynamics that manifest in regard to other forms of human diversity (e.g., diversity of race, culture, gender, or sexual orientation). These dynamics include the dynamics of social power relations—the dynamics of social inequality, privilege, and oppression—as well as the dynamics by which diversity, when embraced, acts as a source of creative potential within a group or society. (Walker, 2021, p. 19-20)

This paradigm challenges us to move beyond a reductive "Well, sure, everyone's different" mindset; instead, the neurodiversity paradigm sees all variation in neurological functioning—not just a few preselected types of variation—as natural and normal but also valuable, worthy of being on the life raft. Along these lines, Ruth Osorio (2021) (she/her pronouns) explores the concept of *disability as insight*, an approach that values disabled perspectives, centers goals of access and accessibility, and positions disability as a vibrant wellspring of wisdom, creativity, and potential. The neurodiversity paradigm also recognizes that social and cultural factors can impact neurodivergence but do not constitute it. That is, our species is naturally neurodiverse. Categorizing some variations of neurodivergence as disordered is oppressive, and attributing more stigma and violence to some than others is cruel.

Throughout this project, I draw several cross- and interdisciplinary connections between writing assessment, composition pedagogy and administration, disability justice, and TPC. These connections offer writing assessment additional research-based avenues to equity and justice, ones where students are the locus of our work. When it comes to writing assessment in classrooms and programs, too few tools are created in concert with students. Instead, there's extensive use of grading schemas and placement processes imposed upon students rather designed with them, and there are widespread models of grading that do harm by limiting the ways in which students can relate to the course material, their peers, their instructor, and their own learning. Justice-oriented writing assessment scholarship has largely interrogated how assessment tools participate in and perpetuate linguistic, racial/ethnic, and class discrimination, as well as the ways in which hegemonic power structures those tools (Poe & Inoue, 2016; Elliot, 2016; Inoue, 2015, 2019). But we're lacking robust models for examining how neuronormativity structures writing pedagogies and assessments (Carillo, 2021; Kryger & Zimmerman, 2020). And though there are recent collaborations tending to issues of social justice in writing assessment at the disciplinary level (such as Gere et al., 2021), there's still space for scholarship and pedagogical practices that help teachers make space for non-normative ways of being and learning. There are a few primary principles that inform and sustain this project. The following sections describe these two principles, which are bolstered by the ten principles of disability justice and the cross-disciplinary connections created throughout the project.

Localization as Connectivity and Community

Localization is a fundamental aspect of both writing assessment and UX design methodologies. In writing assessment scholarship, localization is a process of attunement, a means of ensuring assessments are well-situated within the context of the course, program, unit, or institution in which they operate. In TPC, social justice orientations to localization make arguments to include the populations directly impacted by the technology (Acharya, 2019;

Agboka, 2013). Participatory localization (Agboka, 2013) in particular can be a methodology for centering students' knowledge and experiences in course design, assessment, and placement, and it can help us all develop critical connections and solidarity between students, teachers, staff, and administrators. This approach to localization supports the common disability studies phrase "Nothing about us without us" (Costanza-Chock, 2020b) as well as the disability justice principle of "Leadership of the Most Impacted," which Sins Invalid (2015) explains as "lifting up, listening to, reading, following, and highlighting the perspectives of those who are most impacted by the systems we fight against." It's about centering the needs, goals, and dreams of the stakeholders with the most to lose and the best knowledge of the systems. Localization is a methodology by which writing assessment theory, participatory design, UX, design justice, and disability justice may all converge to accomplish the goal of centering those impacted by our work, valuing and privileging their voices, and attuning to their needs.

Localization will, as a matter of procedure, differ by context. If there's one concept contemporary writing assessment scholars agree on, it's creating locally-based assessments (Adler-Kassner & O'Neill, 2010; O'Neill et al., 2009). This can mean beginning and sustaining the design process locally by involving both students and colleagues and by creating shared language for shared values. But the meaning of local, and location, can also vary by context. Does local mean the students in my class, does it mean the program or unit housing the course, the university community, or the physically local community? In this project, I propose that localization can and should mean all of the above, depending on the purposes of the assessment. I take up the tensions between global vs. local in Chapter 3, where I discuss directed self-placement (DSP) and its need for specific types of localization.

When I dream of a localization, I dream of classrooms based in crip community building: beginning with students. Drawing from the vital work of Piepzna-Samarasinha (2018) in articulating the need for and beauty of "care work," sarah madoka currie and Ada Hubrig (2022) describe crip community building in classrooms as "center[ing] students' needs and the lived expertise of marginalized students before considering institutional expectations, curriculum outcomes, and on-campus mandates" (p. 132). Crip community building asks us to sustain solidarity between students and teachers, rather than adversarial rhetorics and pedagogies, and to build structures that don't leave anyone behind. I dream of educational communities designing documents and classroom procedures that *absorb* labor rather than (re)creating it (currie & Hubrig, 2022). If we design locally and with students involved as the primary stakeholder, these dreams become possibilities.

Radical Trust and Flexibility as Access

The phenomenology of trust—the experience of being trusted and trustworthy, of offering one's trust, of sharing trust and holding it close—has an important role in teaching. It's not always intuitive, either. For me it fluctuates like a barometer (results changing with pressure). On high-anxiety days, for example, I'm not instinctively very trusting of others. It's something I have to consciously consider on days like that, or in situations when I'm stressed. I make this conscious effort to question when/why/how I'm extending or withholding trust because I believe radical trust is a vital component in any writing assessment ecology. This guiding principle of trust is brought to us by adrienne maree brown (2017): "Trust the People. (If you trust the people, they become trustworthy)" (p. 42). I also enjoy this simple directive from Jesse Stommel (2017): "Start by trusting students." It may not seem radical to everyone, but this core principle of trust can be difficult to achieve in an educational culture that literally profits from positioning itself in opposition with or hierarchically to students. As AI writing tools continue improving their capabilities, there will be another influx of technologies that exist purely to look for cheating or plagiarism. At my institution, the lack of trust feels endemic: since the release of ChatGPT, I haven't gone a week without an instructor expressing fear or frustration with the unending laziness of students. As I discuss in Chapter 4, there's no space for this sort of thinking in an assessment ecology that seeks to reduce harm for students.

Flexibility as access is exactly what it says on the tin and more. When I think of access and accessibility, I imagine annoyingly flexible systems, rules, structures—ways of doing the bending and stretching for students, rather than asking them to be perpetually resilient (asking them to endure more, and more, and more). A common example of this is crip time: a transformative and radically flexible approach to normative conceptions of time, temporarily, and timeliness. (A friend of mine likes to say, "Time is a weird soup," and they are correct.) In Tara Wood's (2017) (she/her pronouns) article about crip time in writing classrooms, she suggests paying attention to how time is constructed in our classrooms: not just how much time is allotted per task, but also the structures around and implications of time allocations. Wood writes, "The belief that student writers, given a set amount of time, have an equitable opportunity to perform in a way that suits their cognitive style and pace relies on an assumption of normativity" (2017, p. 269). Often, embracing flexibility requires some degree of letting go of control, and that can be difficult for instructors who have only known white-knuckle pedagogies.

An ethic of flexibility as access wants assessment ecologies that are flexible rather than people who are flexible. This principle follows the "fix systems, not people" (Reed, 2018) premise, one I find crucial to all justice-oriented endeavors. Throughout this dissertation, I argue that flexibility is more than benevolent extensions of empathy or Universal Design for Learning (UDL), it's about being responsive to diverse modes of teaching, learning, and being. It's about deeply trusting students and building structures that trust them, too.

The three body chapters of this dissertation are individual articles. In the following section, I summarize what they seek to accomplish. Each article examines a different assessment site, guided by the principles outlined above, with specific focuses on neuronormativity, localization, and flexibility as care work and a means of access.

Chapter Summaries & Proposed Venues

Chapter 2: Neuronormativity and Validation for Equity

Chapter 2 develops a theoretical understanding of validity from a disability justice perspective. It's shaped to be an article for the *Journal of Writing Assessment* (JWA), which is an open-access journal that frequently publishes equity-oriented scholarship related to writing assessment, and they accept a broad range of qualitative, quantitative, and mixed-methods pieces. This article provides an accessible entry point to conversations about neurodiversity, disability justice, and validity theory. After providing an overview of assessment validity theory, including historical tensions between educational measurement studies and writing assessment, this article contextualizes three models of social-justice oriented validity: consequential validity (Gallagher, 2012; Medina & Walker, 2018), assessment ecologies and racial validity (Inoue, 2009b, 2015), and validity as fairness (Elliot, 2016). I examine the affordances and constraints of these models, paying special attention to the ways they could potentially address aspects of disability and neurodiversity justice. Building on the antiracist assessment scholarship of the last several years (Inoue, 2015, 2019; Poe & Inoue, 2016) and the equity-oriented Fourth Wave of writing assessment (Behm & Miller, 2012), this chapter argues that socially just theories of writing assessment must interrogate and denaturalize neuronormativity (the sticky remnants of the pathology paradigm). In response to these concerns, I end the chapter with a brief call for further examining critical-reflection models of validity and assessment that focuses on community building and flexibility as access.

Chapter 3: Localizing Directed Self-Placement: UX Stories and Methods

Chapter 3 examines directed self-placement (DSP), which is regarded by many as a more inclusive, accessible, and equitable writing placement model than placing students by ACT/SAT exam scores or other single-measurement systems. This article was developed for a special issue of *JWA* on student self-placement (which is currently in process and scheduled for publication in April 2024). I was invited to complete a manuscript for the issue. It will be revised alongside two wonderful colleagues and co-authors (Aly Higgins and Catrina Mitchum) whose work at the intersections of UX and writing placement informed much of this work.

In this article, I argue that technical and professional communication (TPC) and user experience (UX) research methods can integrate equity, engagement, and advocacy into the DSP process by foregrounding accessibility and usability from the beginning. This TPC orientation to DSP offers student-centered method/ologies to develop more precise and equitable localization: the process through which DSP is attuned to its institutional and communal contexts and made relevant to the populations it seeks to serve. I also synthesize the theoretical relations between DSP and TPC (especially regarding models of localization). I follow this discussion of scholarship with storied examples from my institution, providing a sample range of UX methods that (1) are flexible across contexts, (2) are relatively manageable to implement, and (3) are cognizant of WPA, staff, and students' time, labor, and compensation concerns. We know that no assessment technology is in itself socially just and that these systems change over time, and WPAs must be ever vigilant in designing for equity. For DSP, that means the inclusion of placement's key stakeholders—our students. Through UX, we can begin that vital work.

Chapter 4: Depathologizing the Writing Classroom

Chapter 4 examines commonplaces of neuronormativity in composition classrooms and first-year writing pedagogy. Positioned for a journal such as *College English* or *Disability Studies Quarterly*, this article interrogates three deeply embedded nodes of neuronormativity in writing classrooms: Laziness and Procrastination, Time and Control, and Trust and Disclosure. Laziness, for example, is analyzed as an ableist myth. In each of these sections, I use personal and experiential knowledge to illuminate the complexities and interconnectedness of these nodes and their sometimes harmful consequences. Following those analyses, the Implementation section provides practical suggestions for implementing disability justice concepts (such as crip time) and shifting the needle toward crip-community-building pedagogies. Drawing from the ever-expanding confluence of disability studies, composition studies, and writing assessment scholarship, this article seeks to further bridge the gap between theory and practice.

Speed of Trust

I am admittedly still new to many of these ideas. While I am a neurodivergent/disabled student and teacher and can speak from that perspective, disability is not a monolith, and in being White and multiply privileged, I am likely to overlook elements others find crucial. I do hope others take this work and make it better. This labor was one of deep love, frustration, and always-growing notions of crip community building. In considering how to best move forward, I reflect on adrienne maree brown's (2017) recommendation to "move at the speed of trust," (p. 42). I wonder whether I was able to, given the intensive time strictures of this doctoral program, really process my experiences and the research that's been (re)illuminating them. I wonder if I had time to move at the speed of my trust in myself, knowing that time flows differently for me. I know I sometimes outsource my trust to others, soaking up their faith in me to bolster my own. In a beautiful moment of access intimacy, one of the youth athletes I coach at the local climbing gym recently told me, "Believe in the me that believes in you."

I reflect on the "speed of trust" principle also because the time strictures of many classrooms don't facilitate moving at a speed that allows for solidarity building (I.E. communal relationality, care work, or collective access) between students and teachers. It doesn't help that teachers of all kinds are functionally and emotionally overburdened by so many things: state, national, professional, and/or graduate exam requirements, sociocultural/academic expectations, institutional and programmatic assessments, difficult and/or extensive topics in short times, teacher evaluation results, leadership and administrative work, activism and/or community support work, minimal pay, and so on. In many spaces in higher education, teachers who make time for community building or developing radical trust are said to be wasting precious time that should instead be spent on course content.

I often hear this argument against socially just practices: they take too much time. They say it's not because they don't believe in equity, it's because they have too much content to cover, too much to do, and not enough support, so they don't have time to reconfigure an entire course, or assessment system, or assignment sequence. For all overworked and underpaid educators, time is an incredibly precious commodity, and I don't doubt anyone who says they don't have any time to spare: human lives are messy, and U.S. American culture exalts exhaustion. But I do try to encourage them to consider the consequences of *not* making any changes, and to consider what values their current configurations are validating. I ask myself: Am I tacitly implying to my students that they should be as franticly busy as I am? Do my assessments prioritize efficiency and productivity, rather than reflection and deep learning? What can I prioritize instead? How do my evaluative criteria reflect those values? Am I prioritizing "critical connections over critical mass" (brown, 2017, p. 3)? Or am I imagining something entirely different? Importantly: am I doing that imagination work for my students or with them?

As teachers, we're often in positions to leverage power to protect and advocate rather than penalize or police. We're also just as vulnerable to (re)traumatization, ableism, racism, and oppression. Scholars must remember disabled teachers in their work. There's no doubt teaching is difficult work, and it's messy. How we cope with the mess matters, but how we relate to and conceive of the mess is vital too. adrienne maree brown (2017) reminds us that we're in an "imagination battle" (p. 18), arguing that we need radical imagination to inspire, ideate, and enact change. This project seeks to imagine a world where our relationship to assessment as a means of learning is capacious and generative, where our and our students' relationship to learning isn't mediated through the violence of grading, and where teachers are given time and space to move at the speed of trust, whatever that means for them and their students.

Chapter Two

NEURONORMATIVITY
AND VALIDATION FOR EQUITY

When COVID-19 interrupted life as we knew it, the responsiveness of teachers across the world was tremendous. Within a matter of days, teachers had shifted courses to completely online modalities and rearranged all their syllabi and schedules. For many teachers, one of the biggest challenges was assessment: often unquestioned items like attendance, in-class participation, and late policies had to be either seriously overhauled or disregarded entirely. Teachers' priorities, too, underwent massive changes. We were all suddenly less concerned about student "success" and more concerned about student (and instructor/staff) health and safety. Pedagogy suddenly *had* to be humane. Course content that had previously been inaccessible outside the physical classroom was made more widely available than previously thought possible. Accommodation requests (formal accessibility requests requiring diagnoses and disclosure of one's disability) were suddenly widely available everywhere. During those first few months of worldwide quarantine especially, *everything* was online.

In essence, the COVID-19 pandemic stress-tested systems that were built within ableist paradigms, and people with disabilities took note: it was possible to have nationwide and institution-wide change, but it had to be driven by and beneficial to non-disabled people first and foremost. The fact that the results benefited everyone was largely a happy coincidence. The COVID-19 pandemic showed us what is possible when there is collective panic, as well as its inverse, collective action. It also highlighted some of the faulty wiring of the dominant ideologies around ability and disability, especially with teaching and grading.

Many competing ideologies shape our teaching and learning, and we have inherited systems of educational assessment built for the purposes of ranking, sorting, and excluding. Traditionally, students' academic performance is measured against normative standards of learning or "excellence" derived from ableist, White supremacist, and colonialist values. Such assessments are leveraged to advantage certain populations, and they frequently perpetuate structural violence, such as Black students being disproportionately placed in "basic writing" or "developmental" first-year writing courses (Inoue, 2009b; Klausman & Lynch, 2022). This leverage is *structural*, meaning that discrimination emanates from the *design* rather than individual *intent*. That is the main premise of structural violence: there are no clear assailant-victim connections, and it doesn't require intentionality on the part of the assailant (Lederman & Warwick, 2018, p. 233). Instances of structural violence are also not disjunctive; they work in tandem with other systems of oppression. Disability scholars, especially those converging with disability justice activism, critical race theory, and queer/feminist theory, advocate for an intersectional understanding of disability. Structures of power are intricately layered, and their benefits and harms are likewise interlocked (Piepzna-Samarasinha, 2018; Samuels, 2014; Schalk, 2018). Just as there are structural and naturalized race- and class-based assumptions in assessment and placement practices (Gilman et al., 2019; Henson & Hern, 2019; Inoue, 2015; Toth, 2018), there are also able-bodied and pathologizing norms guiding conceptions of writing, reading, and rhetoric (Price, 2011; Smilges, 2021; Yergeau, 2018), constructions of time and timeliness (Wood, 2017), student labor and participation (Carillo, 2021; Kryger & Zimmerman, 2020), and administrative policies (Nicolas, 2017). Disability reaches every level of academia and plays a role in so many layers of writing classrooms, writing centers, and writing programs. Those who operate in these spaces must not let the desire for normalcy countermand all the accessible and humane changes made during the first few terrifying months of COVID-19. As pandemic variants continue developing and spreading, and as social responsivity lessens, it is imperative that we attend to what disability justice advocates have to say about collective access and collective care.

For decades, disability studies research has illuminated the ways in which educational institutional systems are steeped in medical frameworks for diagnosing and treating physical, behavioral, and mental difference, leading to critical analyses of ableist pedagogies and institution-wide lack of awareness accessibility issues (Goodley, 2017). By contrasting the widely accepted pathology paradigm with the neurodiversity paradigm, I offer insight into the ways in which neuronormativity shapes assessment, particularly through concepts of validity. Because it relies on and engenders positivist traditions of assessment, validity is an aspect of assessment ripe for disability justice interventions.

As discussed in Chapter 1, social justice work in writing assessment has so far largely analyzed linguistic, racial, and class-based oppression and how modes of power can structure assessments in those ways. Such scholarship can benefit from disability studies, particularly disability justice, and its deeply intersectional frameworks. Social justice work cannot ignore disability any more than disability can disconnect from racism, colonialism, cisheteropatriarchy, or classism. There is generative potential in disability justice principles of collective access and cross-movement solidarity. Indeed, throughout this dissertation, I contribute to and rely on the rich histories of composition pedagogy, disability studies, and writing assessment scholarship that have come before me, especially those seeking liberatory and equitable practices for both students *and* teachers. I hope to create more pathways in this direction.

Defining Neuronormativity

I mentioned how COVID-19 acted as a sort of "stress test" for ableist paradigms. The global pandemic demonstrated how widespread accommodations were possible, but only with pressure of collective action and threat of widespread death, and only when non-disabled people are at risk. Though COVID-19 shone light on these systemic inequalities and many aspects of their respective paradigms, they're still active. One of the most pervasive ableist paradigms is the pathology paradigm: the set of beliefs that structures society's understanding of the way people think, know, learn, and behave. Nick Walker (she/her pronouns), author of *Neuroqueer Heresies* (2021), explains how the pathology paradigm naturalizes two main assumptions:

1. There is one "right," "normal," or "healthy" way for human brains and human minds to be configured and to function (or one relatively narrow "normal" range into which the configuration and functioning of human brains and minds ought to fall).

2. If your neurological configuration and functioning (and, as a result, your ways of thinking and behaving) diverge substantially from the dominant standard of "normal," then there is Something Wrong With You. (Walker, 2021, p. 18)

The pathology paradigm argues groupings of behaviors and "symptoms" like ADHD and autism are problems to be fixed rather than naturally occurring neurological variation; within this paradigm, my neurodivergent traits are "crippling"—they're just additional hurdles I must clear (or circumnavigate) to proceed along the "normal" path. Many disability scholars refer to these beliefs as aspects of a medical model of disability, which emphasizes curative rhetorics and values (Hamraie, 2017; Linton, 1998). When a faculty member told me that she didn't believe anxiety and depression existed, it was the pathology paradigm giving shape to her worldview. As I discuss more thoroughly in Chapter 4, when students are assumed to be apathetic or recalcitrant for getting distracted in class, for example, the pathology paradigm makes their inattention a matter of character and moral judgment.

No matter its presentation, the results of the pathology paradigm are the same: students (as well as instructors/staff) bear additional burdens *not* because of who they are and/or what they have been through, but because of how our culture structures and treats difference. Educational systems are not built for a diverse student body (Carnevale & Strohl 2013; Johnson, 2022; Naynaha, 2016), especially students *and* faculty/staff with disabilities (Brown & Ramlackhan, 2022; Mellifont, 2021; Merchant et al., 2020; Price, 2011). At present, educational systems operate squarely within the pathology paradigm, and the stakes are increasingly dire. As Hamilton et al. (2021) describe in their research, tuition inflation and increasing costs of education have a disproportionally negative impact on students from historically oppressed groups, low-income families, and/or disability statuses. Students of marginalized/non-normative identities and backgrounds have a fundamentally different experience of higher education than their White, more affluent and normative peers.

If scholarship in placement, retention, and higher education have taught us anything, it is that student pathways matter (Kumar, 2022; Valentine et al., 2017; VanOra, 2019). The systems supposedly bolstering these students must take responsibility for ensuring equitable processes and results. From degree pathways to academic, social, and disability support programs, research suggests that there's a lot more that institutions of higher education can do to create better learning and living conditions for their students (Baik et al., 2019; Koke et al., 2022; Su et al., 2020). Student pathways are often obstructed by barriers like cost, social stigma, lack of awareness, and extracurricular obligations. I once worked with an undergraduate student applying to law school who apologized for yawning because they hadn't slept in two days—they had worked the whole weekend and did coursework and family care in between. When these "new normal" issues are compounded with obstacles related to race/ethnicity, disability, age, gender, sexuality, visa status, level of income, and/or linguistic background, students' academic pathways become unnecessarily complex and outright dangerous to student wellbeing. Assessment at every level of academic institutions impacts student pathways, and the directional forces they exert are still being mapped. These and other barriers to student pathways demonstrate a need for a paradigm that recognizes and redresses these obstructions to student equity, success, and wellbeing.

The directional forces of neuronormativity keep us from questioning what's considered natural/normal and who has deemed it so. Swimming against a current, or even pausing to question the current, is more effortful than going with the flow of the sociopolitical waters around us. Ahmed (2017) contends that *directionality* is a mode of power: if systems of power can predetermine our habits, our thoughts, and our goals in a certain direction, they can maintain a certain level of concealment and control. Lederman and Warwick (2018) argue that assessment is related to structural violence through representation and normativity. For them, assessment is an institutional representation of the student, and the institution rewards proximity to norms and punishes distance from them (p. 250). Assessments have directional power: they can send students down wrong pathways, provide shortcuts, or create roadblocks. Though "invisible," norms are as impactful as physical barriers, as weighty as lodestones, as tall as brick walls. Normativity is both structured and structuring; norms govern social and academic pathways even when they cannot be seen or touched. Alternative paradigms—alternate ways of thinking, valuing, being, doing—are crucial to any project of liberation, and Walker's (2021) answer to the pathology paradigm is the *neurodiversity paradigm.*

At its simplest, the neurodiversity paradigm supports the belief that there is no one correct way to exist, think, or behave. Walker summarizes it in three points:

1. Neurodiversity—the diversity among minds—is a natural, healthy, and valuable form of human diversity.

2. There is no "normal" or "right" style of human mind, any more than there is one "normal" or "right" ethnicity, gender, or culture.

3. The social dynamics that manifest in regard to neurodiversity are similar to the social dynamics that manifest in regard to other forms of human diversity (e.g., diversity of race, culture, gender, or sexual orientation). These dynamics include the dynamics of social power relations—the dynamics of social inequality, privilege, and oppression—as well as the dynamics by which diversity, when embraced, acts as a source of creative potential within a group or society. (Walker, 2021, p. 19-20)

This paradigm positions neurological variation as a natural and valuable aspect of human diversity rather than as "mental disorders" like those classified by the DSM-5 and ICD-11.[7] Unlike the pathology paradigm, which views my neurodivergence as a sickness to be cured or a personal failing, the neurodiversity paradigm views my anxiety and ADHD as aspects of my unique neurological build, as two lines of the fingerprint of my mind. This paradigm also recognizes that social and cultural factors can certainly impact neurodivergence but do not constitute it. That is, our species is naturally neurodiverse. Categorizing certain neurological variations as disordered (some with far more stigma than others) is a form of oppression that has widespread and devastating consequences.

---

[7] Respectively, the American Psychiatric Association's (2013) *Diagnostic and Statistical Manual of Mental Disorders* (5th ed.; DSM-5) and the World Health Organization's (2019) *International Statistical Classification of Diseases and Related Health Problems* (11th ed.; ICD-11).

Within the pathology paradigm, many ableist norms govern our patterns of behavior, our thinking, and our opinions of ourselves and others. This is neuronormativity: the package of rules that substantiate and maintain the pathology paradigm. Normativity is what helps naturalize and neutralize aspects of any given paradigm. As Sara Ahmed (2017) (she/her pronouns) reminds us, "We cannot 'not' live in relation to norms" (p. 43); and as Walker (2021) explains, building upon the foundational work of Audre Lorde, "The task of liberating ourselves from the master's house begins with dismantling the parts of that house that have been built within our own heads" (p. 26). When norms are denaturalized and questioned, the paradigm can slip, deteriorate, destabilize. When I use the word "neuronormativity," I mean to reference the ways in which normativity is embedded within and substantiates the pathology paradigm.

Though Walker uses this word on occasion in her work, my understanding of the term came about with my initial discomfort with (and some ignorance about) "neurotypical," which I had understood as implying an untroubled binary of *divergent* and *typical*. Walker (2021) argues that "neurotypical" and "neurodivergent" are in fact opposites, as straight is to queer (p. 40). But I wanted a word to discuss the specific norms of the pathology paradigm without having to associate all my observations and analyses with neurotypicality. Thus, *neuronormativity* allows me to identify areas between neurotypicality and the norms that undergird the pathology paradigm, so as to not conflate the two. Throughout this dissertation, this word will *not* replace the word neurotypical; instead, it will be used in places where I am referencing norms of the pathology paradigm. I will use the word "neurotypical" when referring to someone or something that exists comfortably in the pathology paradigm, rather than the norms that constitute it.

The word "neuroqueer" also has salience in these conversations. Like its eponymous relative *queer*, neuroqueer denotes an active resistance, subversion, or otherwise queering of both neuronormativity and cis/allo/heteronormativity. While it can be an adjective and thus a social identity, neuroqueering also seeks to address or interrupt intersectional oppression of queerness and neurodivergence. As Walker succinctly puts it, "One can neuroqueer, and one can be neuroqueer" (2021, p. 161). When exploring the intersections of neurodivergence and queerness, or perhaps their mutuality and inseparability, or perhaps their overlapping oppressions, one can use the word "neuroqueer" to suggest both/either the social identity and/or the act of neuroqueering.

There are certainly many connections between composition pedagogy and disability studies, especially since the publication of *Disability and the Teaching of Writing: A Critical Sourcebook* (Lewiecki-Wilson & Brueggemann, 2008). While scholars have written about how assessment structures pathways by race, ethnicity, class, gender, and linguistic resources, we are lacking in studies that examine the ways in which assessment structures opportunities for disabled students, many of whom are multiply disabled or multiply oppressed, whose multidimensional lives exist beyond the seemingly infinitely divisible nature of social categories. In the sections below, I provide a brief history of composition and assessment to highlight the incongruous nature of educational measurement and writing assessment pursuits, and then I analyze three types of validity: consequential validity, racial validity, and fairness as validity. These models of validity are unified by their efforts toward equity in writing assessment (specifically by examining the larger value systems in addition to the methodological bits and bobs). From this work, I suggest an approach to validity that prioritizes the principles and aims of disability justice.

Contextualist Paradigm of Assessment

Writing assessment in the United States developed alongside 19th-century literacy crises and, a little later, concerns for validating the use of student writing to evaluate student academic preparedness (with "students" denoting wealthy White men of primarily European descent). Since the inclusion of composition into Harvard's college entrance exams in 1874, student writing in American institutions has been inextricably bound to concerns of not just academic preparedness but also professional preparedness, resulting in emphases on efficiency, grammar, and surface-level correctness (Brereton, 1995; Crowley, 1998). To contextualize this period in American history: slavery had been abolished for only about ten years; women wouldn't have the right to vote for roughly fifty more years (with Black women facing substantially more obstacles to voting until the Civil Rights Movement and the passage of the Voting Rights Act of 1965; see Jones, 2020); legislation granting Indigenous peoples American citizenship wouldn't be passed until 1924; many Ivy League schools wouldn't admit women until the 1960's (Malkiel, 2016); and the Individuals with Disabilities Education Act (previously "Education for All Handicapped Children Act") wouldn't be enacted until 1975. Though there were women's colleges and Black colleges by this time, the foundations of educational measurement and writing assessment were largely developed by wealthy non-disabled White men of the professoriate.

On the heels of shifting social and professional landscapes, American universities developed composition courses as a means of educating those who were "lacking" in current American academic English. As a result, "good writing became narrowly defined as error-free writing" (Adler-Kassner & O'Neill, 2010, p. 45). Entrance exams and composition courses needed to be scaled to serve increasing (and increasingly diverse) student populations, and industrialist/modernist emphases on efficiency and objectivity resulted in "universal" evaluative measures such as standardized writing exams. As Adler-Kassner and O'Neill (2010) usefully summarize, the standardization of college entrance exams exemplifies the values of positivism and capitalism that would give way to the development of psychometrics and would influence the field of educational measurement up to present day. Yancey (1999), Huot (2002), and others (Adler-Kassner & O'Neill, 2010; Lynne, 2004) discuss how the overlapping interests of educational measurement and writing studies have contributed to the history of writing assessment *and* vice versa (Elliot, 2015)—writing is so frequently used as a means of assessment that it cannot be ignored by the field of educational measurement. While we still rely on concepts from educational measurement and psychometrics, Lynne (2004) argues writing assessment must forge its own path and develop its own theory of assessment outside the realm of objectivist, positivist paradigms. She explains how validity in particular is a word that "characterize[s] writing assessment as a technical activity with objective outcomes" rather than a complex socially situated rhetorical activity (p. 3). In *Coming To Terms: A Theory of Writing Assessment*, Lynne (2004) reasons through a contextualist paradigm of assessment, one that is responsive to the values and expertise of teachers and scholars of rhetoric and composition studies. In place of validity and reliability, she offers the words "meaningful" and "ethical" respectively (p. 117), arguing that these terms bring the theorizing of writing assessment into the realm of composition, making it easier to situate the process within social constructivist epistemologies that align with contemporary composition praxes.

In recent years, Asao B. Inoue, a leading scholar in antiracist writing assessment and writing program administration, has also shifted to more compositionist-friendly terminology. Although "validity" and "reliability" have the potential to be useful, Inoue notes, "A different set of accessible terms are needed for teachers and students. ... old psychometric terms can be a barrier for many teachers to thinking carefully about classroom writing assessment because most are not familiar with them and many see them connected to positivistic world views about language and judgment" (2015, p. 13). Shifting toward language that resonates with writing studies practitioners can be a valuable exercise in iterative design and feedback loops, which is a staple of writing assessment theory. Refining terminology through localization can mean (re)articulating values, questioning purposes, and examining the "system" itself. Such reflexivity can also illuminate patterns of structural violence, such as institutional racism. Reconciling the positivist echoes of educational management in writing assessment is not finished, especially as disciplinary and pedagogical values continue expanding to incorporate aims of antiracist and disability justice. In the rest of this chapter, I take a closer look at three promising areas of writing assessment and validity development: consequential validity, racial validity, and fairness in validity. These three areas have much to teach us about the current state of writing assessment theory and its potential for disability justice interventions.

Examining Validity

Validity, like its sister concept reliability, is a keystone of assessment and research. In writing assessment and beyond, there are several definitions and approaches to validation, many of which offer perspectives on different aspects of the assessment/research process. For decades, there was a "holy trinity" (Guion, 1980) model of validity:

1. Criterion validity: correlation to external criteria (I.E. Can the GRE predict how well a person will do in graduate school? Does it accurately measure preparedness?)

2. Content validity: the domain of knowledge, ability, or trait being measured (I.E. Do the questions in the GRE accurately evaluate knowledge of certain subject areas?)

3. Construct validity: the *construct* or the theoretical conception of the thing being measured (I.E. How is "preparedness" conceived of in the GRE? How does this understanding of "preparedness" influence the exam's design, implementation, results, and consequences? How narrowly or broadly is "preparedness" conceived and measured?)

These three aspects of validity were frequently used piecemeal rather than as a unified system (Huot, 2002), resulting in validity being largely reduced to the latter—construct validity and its theoretical legacy, the "argument-based approach to [test] validation" (Kane, 2013). This model is now generally referred to as the "validity argument approach" and recognizes that it must "unify assessment design, interpretation, use, and validation" (Dorsey & Michaels, 2022). Built upon this argument-approach bedrock, the *Standards for Educational and Psychological Testing* (American Educational Research Association, American Psychological Association, & National Council on Measurement in Education, 2014) defines validity as the "degree to which evidence and theory support the interpretations of test scores for proposed uses of tests" (p. 11). This definition has a long history of revisions, as Elliot (2015) usefully catalogs, and this most recent revision attempts to grapple with fairness by placing it alongside validity and reliability/precision as part of an overall process of assessment design.

In a more recent articulation of validity, Robert J. Mislevy (2018, 2021) argues for a "sociocognitive" approach to educational measurement based on contemporary research from "cognitive science, social psychology, linguistics, and many other fields" (2021, p. 56). He argues that assessment for writing specifically ought to be viewed as "evidentiary argument, situated in social contexts, centered on students' developing competences in valued activities, and shaped by purposes and values—chief among them validity, fairness, and opportunity to learn" (p. 54). He also notes, "The matchup between an assessment and its uses determines its usefulness, validity, and fairness" (p. 58), further suggesting such "uses" must be made explicit. Mislevy concludes by asserting, "Validity and fairness originate in conception and design, before the first data point appears" (p. 66). He thus advocates for an assessment model that aligns more readily with a contextualist paradigm outlined by Lynne (2004) and others, though his emphasis remains on "use arguments" and other psychometric terminology and touchstones.

I begin with this scholarship from the field of educational measurement for several reasons: (1) to show how writing assessment has long been (and will likely continue to be) in conversation with this and many other fields of study; (2) to show that concepts of validity have shifted over time as paradigms and sociocultural landscapes have shifted; (3) to show that many of the assessment concepts we draw on today have few contemporary adaptations. Elliot (2015) reminds us, "If there is a single instrumental lesson to be learned from the past, it is that interpretation and impact are historically contingent and inextricably bound" (p. 678). Validity is not an immutable holdover from bygone eras, though it is perhaps resistant to change (like many institutional foundations). This brief interdisciplinary overview helps to contextualize the writing assessment approaches to validity I will examine shortly.

In writing assessment specifically, the commonplace definition of validity is often phrased as a question: "Does this assessment item (rubric, test, etc.) measure what it seeks or professes to measure?" Our sources for this definition are Edward White (1994) and Kathleen Yancey (1999), though our more robust articulations of validity are developed primarily from the work of Kane (2006; 2013) and Messick (1989a; 1989b; 1995) and many others in educational measurement (Guion, 1977; Mislevy, 2021). Norbert Elliot explains some of this history in his article "Validation: The Pursuit," and he also describes the ways in which validity has taken such precedence in assessment conversations. He writes, "the concepts [of validity/certainty] adapt equally well—so well that we may wonder if they are not merely artifacts of the system but, rather, the System itself" (Elliot, 2015, p. 669). Ellen Cushman (2016) (she/her pronouns) expands on this claim, arguing that validity is both a tenet and a tool, making it particularly difficult to deconstruct: it is both a technology and an ideology, both the bricks and the brick masons. As a foundation of modern institutions rooted in imperialism, capitalism, and the industrial revolution, validity "indicates the social and epistemic hierarchies of knowledge created as part of the colonial difference. What is deemed to be valid in arguments and therefore reliably consistent in its measures needs the necessary other of the invalid and unreliable to legitimize themselves" (Cushman, 2016). The evaluation and categorization of disabilities, especially mental disabilities, have historically rendered disabled folks unreliable, invalid, and untrustworthy, damning them to the peripheries of society (especially if they're connected to another historically marginalized group/identity). Concepts of validity undergird all health disorder diagnostic criteria and processes, especially those of mental "disorders" (a term that functionally signifies the pathology paradigm) and are thus extremely relevant to disability justice communities. But in the realm of writing assessment, validity holds many implications for teachers, students, and administrators: institutions demand the validation of programmatic operations, students want valid grades and placements, and teachers want to ensure their grading practices aren't doing more harm than good.

Understanding of validity hasn't strayed far from White and Yancey's early articulation of it, at least not in common discourse. For my purposes in this chapter, rather than offering another definition of validity, I want to linger on Cushman's (2016) entreaty:

The important thing is actively seeking out pluriversal (rather than universal) understandings, multiple and varied (rather than singular and narrow) ways of expression, integrated (rather than siloed) exercises in validity and reliability, whole and active

(rather than atomized and static) language uses in an effort to name and respect a range of

ontological, axiological, and epistemological perspectives.

The three types of validity I explore and analyze below offer both methodological heuristics as

well as systems-level inquiries—rather than fixating simply on the tools or assessment

technologies at play, these models inquire into the broader value systems that structure our

commonplace assumptions about writing assessment.

Consequential Validity

Consequential validity asks us to attune to and validate the consequences of a given

assessment. Cruz Medina and Kenneth Walker's (2018) description resonates with disability

justice principles (Sins Invalid, 2015, 2019): "Consequential validity is an inquiry framework

that uses explicit values to interrogate the potential and current effects of our pedagogy for all

students, but in this case, particularly for systemically marginalized students" (p. 47). With this

definition, they recognize "potential and current effects," which grounds users in the present and

also maintains space for future consequentiality; just as described by Sins Invalid (2015), Medina

and Walker also recognize that marginalized students ought to be centered in efforts to improve

assessment and pedagogical praxes. In their chapter, they describe how they incorporate

consequential validity into their technical and professional writing courses from an explicitly

social-justice framework. For Medina and Walker, consequential validity for classroom

assessment is about making course values and expectations explicit, and it's about making space

for student resistance, potentiality/emergence, and the interrogation of power relations (2018, p.

52-53). Their approach doesn't seek to silence students with grades, to erase difference, or to eliminate all conflict. Medina and Walker's emphasis on transparency, flexibility, and critical frameworks shows how models of validity can be repurposed for the goals of equity and justice.

In other articulations, consequential validity arose in response to the traditional psychometric uses of validity outlined above. In Chris W. Gallagher's (2012) understanding, consequential validity attempts to move away from outcomes-based assessment, which has a functionally limited scope: as end points articulated from the outset, outcomes can detract from emergent, unpredictable factors arising in the development and usage of the assessment. In short, consequences of an assessment often disrupt or displace intended outcomes. For Gallagher (2012), consequential validity aims to do three main things:

1. Contextualize assessment goals without disregarding disciplinary standards;

2. Engage with those external disciplinary standards without inflexible adherence; and

3. Make programmatic space for "emerging, unintended, and perhaps highly significant consequences" of assessments. (p. 56)

These objectives thus shift the focus of the assessment to purposes and impact. Other authors have also explicitly promoted consequential validity, such as Lee J. Cronbach (1998) and Brian Huot (2002), and their work informed that of Gallagher (2012) and, more recently, Medina and Walker (2018). Others have folded consequentiality concerns into their assessment system without naming it as such, particularly in placement assessment. Taken together, the body of scholarship around consequential validity demonstrates the importance of going beyond outcomes-first assessments, beyond simply validating for rigid objectives, and instead looking at the potentiality of the entire context and all its brilliant complexities.

With Medina and Walker's (2018) version of consequential validity, the flow of power dynamics in the classroom is intentionally paused, not by the assessment tool (rubric, grading contract, etc.), but by the manner in which they implemented their localized grading contracts and the specific emphases they placed on student involvement. As I have argued elsewhere (Kryger & Zimmerman, 2020) and discuss further in Chapter 4, the existence of an equity-minded assessment tool accomplishes very little toward those aims if the person(s) or system(s) implementing the tool do not identify with the values and goals informing it. As Lederman and Warwick (2018) further explain, we sometimes take for granted the site-based, locally-controlled, and context-sensitive nature of writing assessment, which is a very different context than educational measurement, which largely deals with tests designed to be used across many contexts. It makes sense that writing studies would move toward a consequentiality-based model of validation, since we are deeply concerned with the impacts of our assessments. But from disability justice and neurodiversity paradigm frameworks, there must also be components of relational accountability, flexibility, and accessibility built into the analyses of consequentiality and the uptake of the results of those analyses, not just localization (the process of attuning an assessment to its local context). This means students (especially non-White, disabled, queer, trans, and multiply marginalized students) have an active seat at that table and their input isn't just heard, it's valued. Any analysis of the consequential validity of classroom writing assessment will not be complete without consulting those intended to benefit from the evaluation of their learning and without honoring the relationships forged through its implementation.

Racial Validity

Racial validity is a means of validating assessment technologies through the categories of Power, Parts, and Purpose (Inoue, 2009b), a heuristic Asao B. Inoue (he/him pronouns) later revised in his book *Antiracist Writing Assessment Ecologies: Teaching and Assessing Writing for a Socially Just Future* (2015). Racial validity offers a means of analyzing assessment systems and data from a critical and ecological heuristic, including the analysis of individual assessments, their consequences, and their underlying systems of hegemony. While Inoue specifically focuses on "racial formations" (see Omi & Winant, 1994) as the locus of his analyses, racial validity offers a critical lens that can be applied to other social categories of difference and the hegemonic forces that benefit from and sustain them. In essence, antiracist ecologies ask us to consider the entire assessment picture, including the histories, social environments, purposes, communities, and relationships engaged with the development and implementation of the assessment. As Inoue (2009) explains, "Assessment is not a value-free technology because it is more than the methods, machines, and materials we use to make judgments" (p. 101). This initial heuristic and line of thinking contributed directly to the development of Inoue's antiracist and ecological understanding of writing assessment (2015), which remains one of the most extensive and holistic treatments of power, White supremacy, and assessment in the field. Inoue's (2015) assessment ecology model describes seven consubstantial elements for analysis and reflection: Power, Purposes, Places, People, Processes, Parts, and Products (p. 176). In his words, "Writing assessment ecologies are complex systems, resisting simple explanations and visual representations. Ecologies are more than visual. More than textual" (p. 176).

Though Inoue later gave up the phrase "racial validity" in favor of less psychometric terminology (2015, p. 13), his initial treatment of validity is useful for the critical analysis of hegemonic power systems. If, as Inoue deftly demonstrates, racial formations are constructed through assessment technologies, other social categories of difference (such as disability) are also constructed in this way. Inoue's antiracist ecological model of assessment features heuristics that are purposefully applicable across assessment contexts. Disaggregating data by social categories to examine racial validity has been an increasingly popular and useful practice. Disparate impact analysis methodologies, for example, disaggregate such data for legally protected populations (see Poe et al., 2014). In my experience as a writing program placement administrator, I have seen how disaggregation of first-year composition placement data by race and ethnicity can reveal patterns of both systemic and internalized White supremacy. Overall, Inoue's work provides a solid and generative foundation for dreaming of and creating more equitable writing assessments. Though some of his work relies on ideas of student labor, time, and effort that may disadvantage some disabled students, especially neurodivergent students (Carillo, 2021; Kryger & Zimmerman, 2020), Inoue's work on assessment ecologies and racial validity is useful for disability justice in assessment by demonstrating how systems of oppression impact assessment communities.

Fairness in Validity

The last of these three frameworks of validity is Norbert Elliot's (2016) (he/him pronouns) theory of ethics for writing assessment. His theory consists of three main components:

- Maximum construct representation (MCR). MCR can be defined as the broadening of assessment constructs, those theoretical understandings of the relevant evaluative criteria, to their largest operational capacity. For example, integrating broad and pluriversal understandings of what constitutes "good writing," rather than a narrow conception of writing as error-free, when creating evaluative criteria;

- Fairness, which is defined as the structuring of opportunity; and

- Involvement of internal and external stakeholders.

In Elliot's model of fairness for assessment, validity is not situated as a separate endeavor to be initiated when convenient; instead, validity and reliability are unified into a single theory of ethics in which MCR, fairness, and involvement lessen potential inequities. As Elliot explains it, construct *under*representation is the "enemy of valid assessment" because narrow or (de)limited constructs contribute to the absence of fairness in assessment, resulting in the exclusion of historically marginalized groups (2016, p. 6). By implementing broader understandings of constructs, we make space for a more diverse and holistic articulation of assessment criteria.

Elliot proposes assessments that are "construct-rich" (the opposite of construct underrepresentation) and deeply contextualized and that also attend to concerns of fairness *first*. This design protocol subordinates traditional understandings of validity and reliability and recognizes that their operational definitions may shift as the aims and needs of fairness shift over time. Elliot's theory of ethics attempts to attune to ethical uses of assessments, and he situates his work between theories of ethics (Rawls, 1999, 2001), educational measurement, and college writing assessment. In his model, Elliot articulates the importance of facilitating "opportunities to learn" (Gee, 2008), which he sees as critically integrated with MCR—writing pedagogy that, similarly to UDL, expands to meet the most oppressed students' needs.

While MCR is one method of potentially achieving socially just assessment goals, it cannot be the only pathway. As Elliot realizes, there must be a collaborative component to the validation and usage of assessment systems. But in addition to involvement from various internal and external stakeholders, including students, there must also be regular analyses of who benefits from assessment projects and how. Alfie Kohn (2012) and Lederman and Warwick (2018) argue that assessment (especially grading) can harm students. Disability justice advocates for *leadership of the most impacted*, which positions those who best understand the oppressive forces as leaders in projects. The inclusion of students in the development of assessments will continue to be imperative for equity-oriented administrative work.

Neuroqueering Validity

In the broader scope of academia, validity is more like an amulet to ward against inferior research design, implementation, and data/results interpretation. In mixed methods research, for example, validity involves "strategies that address potential threats to drawing correct inferences and accurate assessments from the integrated data" (Creswell & Plano Clark, 2018, p. 251). Creswell and Plano Clark identify over 20 "validity threats" to certain types of research projects, and they offer "strategies to minimize threats" (p. 251). They also describe how some researchers in mixed methods argue for other terms, such as "legitimation" or "inference quality" (p. 250), to get at what they mean by "validity" with more precision. Validity in research methods is discussed in terms of legitimacy, "threats," and viability: its likelihood of getting published, of having its methods reproduced or cited, of being able to share data and analyses with confidence, of contributing to goals of graduating, procuring employment, and/or securing tenure. This academic/researcher/statistician approach to validity strikes me as a "necessary evil": a means of protection from things like inhumane feedback practices, potential loss of grant funding, and scientific skeptics. When the work has been validated, who can question it?

In composition pedagogy, validity can serve more of the purpose Lynne (2004) imagined: a reminder of the *meaningfulness* of assessment, like the "So What?" we sometimes ask our students. Rather than conceiving of validity as protection from external forces, I'm more concerned with the following:

- How teachers make judgments about concepts such as "good" writing, rhetorically "successful" texts, critical thinking, timeliness, and labor;

- How teachers recognize, articulate, and assess (make explicit, rather than tacit) the values of writing in their field/discipline; and

- How teachers can structure assessments that don't rely on or perpetuate naturalized White supremacy, racism, ableism, classism, monolingualism, sexism, queerphobia, transphobia, xenophobia, and/or colonialism.

Building from Lederman and Warwick (2018), the structural violence of assessment must be made explicit, and we must create assessments that actively seek to disrupt structural violence and inequity. From the three types of validity explained above, there are opportunities for expanding upon equity and justice orientations to assessment and validity. Medina and Walker's (2018) version of consequential validity demonstrates how integration with liberatory pedagogies can facilitate justice-minded improvements in classroom assessment. Inoue's (2015) antiracist ecology model provides an overarching heuristic for the analysis and development of assessment systems and their contexts, a model that is responsive to power dynamics, social categories of difference, and ecological, contextual, and local factors. Elliot's (2016) theory of ethics and MCR is likewise useful for moving beyond narrow, neuronormative conceptions of writers, writing, classroom behavior, and course engagement. Each of these three approaches centers fairness from the outset, making social justice the necessary beginning point of their design, implementation, and iteration.

Beyond these versions, validity for writing assessment can also be conceived of as critical reflection. Brian Huot (2002) (he/him pronouns) makes this argument in *(Re)Articulating Writing Assessment for Teaching and Learning*, where he draws on the work of Moss (1998),

Bourdieu and Wacquant (1992), and Cherryholmes (1988). In considering ways of aligning teaching and assessing, Huot writes, "I think it's possible and potentially very beneficial to view validity not as some pronouncement of approval but rather as an ongoing process of critical reflection" (p. 51). He goes on to quote Moss (1998): "validity is a way that 'the inquiry lens is turned back on the researchers and program developers themselves as stakeholders, encouraging critical reflection about their own theories and practices'" (2002, p. 51). What could that look like? Ideally, it looks like relational, flexible, communal, recursive, accessible, and explicitly articulated assessment design, implementation, and iteration. As Gere et al. (2021) articulate, "As a structural matter, justice can be understood as something we partly make and remake through the relationships we inhabit and reinforce; justice, in other words, is the product of justicing" (p. 386–387). It is a matter of reflective, recursive doing. Gere et al. (2021) call for communal justicing, or the active involvement of not just local agents but also folks invested in structural changes at national and disciplinary levels.

While this recommendation is an admirable step forward, Walker (2021) explains how neuronormativity is as pervasive as cisheteronormativity and is thus deeply internalized and embodied (and performative), even by those who are neurodivergent (p. 180). For example, take the commonplace issue of tardiness. The dominant narrative around tardiness is that students are lazy, disrespectful, and/or "bad" students (perhaps even "bad" people). Even disregarding that often students are commuting from great distances on and off campus, as well as the limited "breaks" between class periods, the assumption that students who are late are automatically worse students (or people) than those who are punctual is an ableist assumption rooted squarely in the pathology paradigm: if one cannot functionally exist in the normative time strictures of the academic institution (let alone the rest of the world), there is *Something Wrong With You*. That wrongness is then reflected in institutional and social directionality—it's given physical and emotional shape and manifests as student pathways with additional challenges. And yet some teachers still deduct grade points for students who are late to class, basing their justification of this assessment of student performance and engagement on strict adherence to ableist constructions of time. Because of its neutral and naturalized embeddedness, there is a great deal of academic "performance" around neuronormativity that pervades classroom activity systems, which I discuss in Chapter 4.

I argue for the shifting of validity toward a model of critical reflection, one that incorporates awareness of and accountability to the broader assessment ecology (Inoue, 2015), seeks to actively disrupt social inequity from the beginning and with the intention of doing so (Elliot, 2016; Lederman & Warwick, 2018), and understands its own meaningfulness (Lynne, 2004). This meaningfulness should be localized: co-constructed alongside students to reflect the local communities of practice and not just the values of the institution. By iteratively attuning to communal accountability and pluriversal accounts of assessment, we can make critical space for a wide range of ways of doing, being, and knowing.

Conclusion

As a graduate student administrator, I have learned that the role of the writing program administrator (WPA) requires managing widespread misinformation, expectations, and constraints that are often antithetical to writing studies' values, expertise, and disciplinary knowledge. WPAs are constantly forced to straddle the line between what research shows is best for students' development and the institution's assumptions about assessment, which are often framed through various psychometric theories. My experience working on a multi-university written communication assessment project this past year has solidified my understanding that assessment at the broader institutional level remains woefully behind any of the emergent scholarship happening in either educational measurement *or* writing assessment. As Huot (2002) notes, "assessment procedures that attempt to fix objectively a student's ability to write are based upon an outdated theory supported by an irrelevant epistemology" (p. 94). Do our current writing assessment paradigms really align with our pedagogical values? Often, in practice, no. But within these tensions, we can make space for generative conversations, new methodologies, and even strength of conviction toward resistance. Assessment is, like research, an institutional site that carries with it a great deal of historical and structural race-based and ability-based oppression. But throwing assessment out completely is neither a feasible or worthwhile goal (not presently, anyway). There are strong arguments for self-assessment, which is foundational to directed self-placement (Chapter 3) and some ungrading methodologies (Chapter 4).

In sum, an understanding of validity as critical reflection, supported by communal and ecological accountability, with the aim of interrupting structural violence, is a step we need toward reckoning with the underlying ableism and neuronormativity embedded in assessment systems. If we can reshape how we approach assessment questions about the quality and success of student writers and their writing, we can better situate our assessment practices within the local contexts of all our students and their varied, emergent needs.

Chapter Three

LOCALIZING DIRECTED SELF-PLACEMENT:
UX STORIES AND METHODS

As colleges and universities across the United States seek more efficient, user-friendly, and publicly demonstrable responses to increasingly diverse student populations and demands for equity and inclusion, writing program administrators (WPAs) must examine placement processes for incoming students. The demand for equitable administrative practices must include student self-placement, which I refer to as directed self-placement (DSP). For placement, the stakes are high: research suggests that students' first year courses are an important factor in student success and persistence (Poe et al., 2019). These placement assessments also have a powerful directionality component, as they funnel students in to (or out of) certain course sequences and the pathways beyond. To ensure all students have the broadest possible range of choices and best design for well-informed guidance, we must consider students' experiences with DSP not just in aggregate but also at the personal level. Technical and professional communication (TPC) standards and user experience (UX) design methodologies can help us integrate equity, engagement, and empowerment in our DSP systems by foregrounding accessibility and usability from the beginning. This TPC orientation to DSP offers student-centered design method/ologies for WPAs to develop more precise and equitable DSP localization: the process through which DSP is attuned to its institutional and communal contexts and made relevant to the populations it seeks to serve.

As part of the Fourth Wave of writing assessment scholarship (Behm & Miller, 2012), scholarship has prioritized concerns of assessment equity and fairness, and this social justice orientation has extended to DSP. In particular, DSP has potential as an antiracist assessment practice by facilitating more equitable distributions of racial formations in course enrollments (Inoue, 2009b; Klausman & Lynch, 2022). This means students have open access to all the courses available to them and can self-assess and self-select. For WPAs, students are not only the locus of placement work, they're also the population most highly impacted by the design and outcomes. The stakes are increasingly high: developmental education scholarship shows that students placed in developmental courses/sequences are more likely to never finish their initial coursework or persist to degree (Adams et al., 2009; Valentine et al., 2017), especially in community college contexts (VanOra, 2019). Transfer students also face several unique challenges with placement, credit articulation, and retention (Grites, 2013; Rosenberg, 2016), and students from historically marginalized backgrounds face many additional barriers. WPAs can better support student self-efficacy through more localized, accessible, and usable designs (not just localized content) and equitable representation from all student groups. In other words, through UX, we can both improve literacy-related DSP content *and* improve the design of the placement system. We know from both TPC scholarship (Dorpenyo, 2022) and digital rhetorics (Miller-Cochran & Rodrigo, 2009) that design elements have crucial implications for user engagement and empowerment.

Localization is a fundamental aspect of both writing assessment and UX design methodologies. In writing assessment scholarship, localization is considered a process of attunement, a means of ensuring assessments are well-situated within the context of the class, program, unit, or institution in which the assessment operates. In TPC, localization has a slightly different connotation. According to the Society for Technical Communication (2016), localization is the process of "Creating or customizing a product or service for a specific regional or local market," suggesting that the industry standard regards localization not only as contextualization but also as a means of ensuring usability within (and sometimes across) cultural contexts. In TPC, more recent social justice orientations to localization argue for including the populations directly impacted (Acharya, 2019; Agboka, 2013). In particular, Godwin Agboka's (2013; 2014) (he/him pronouns) framework of participatory localization advocates (1) a dynamic understanding of localization, one that moves beyond linguacultural aspects, and (2) for the co-development of technical communication products alongside users rather than relying on generalized and decontextualized assumptions of users' needs. For placement assessment, which is most certainly a site of social justice, UX method/ologies are a practical and feasible first step toward participatory localization goals.

Though we now have several contextualized examples of DSP implementation (see Nastal et al., 2022), there is little published scholarship directly addressing how to localize for DSP beyond choosing a hosting site, tool design, and crafting questionnaires that address the writing program's learning outcomes. More resources are needed to support DSP localization and its inherent complexities. By describing the process and the results of UX method/ologies for iterating on an existing DSP, this article begins addressing this need. In particular, we explain how the alignment of UX method/ologies and disability justice improves DSP localization. The better we understand our students and their needs, the more accessible and usable our designs will be. This framework also begins addressing Gere et al.'s (2021) call for communal justicing, an approach that aims to disrupt inequities at the disciplinary level by prioritizing structural interventions that include everyone, not just administrators. Especially in writing assessment and placement, trusting our students is imperative, and we can further build and exercise that dialogic trust through UX and participatory localization.

In this article, I provide the theoretical relations between DSP and TPC as well as between writing assessment and TPC models of localization. I follow these discussions with DSP iteration examples from my local institution, providing a sample range of UX methods that (1) are flexible across contexts, (2) are relatively manageable to implement, and (3) are cognizant of both WPA and student time, labor, and compensation concerns. As with writing assessment writ large, there are no panacea UX method/ologies, but these options afford DSP developers the flexibility needed for communal localization.[8] Placement assessment is messy, and UX is messy, but the work is absolutely necessary.

DSP Validity & Efficacy

As a form of assessment, writing placement systems are often beholden to concerns of validity and reliability. Since the inception of college entrance exams and composition courses, placement and its consequences have been a concern of educational measurement and eventually composition studies and writing assessment (Crowley, 1998; Yancey, 1999), with placement trends ranging from holistic essay scoring (White, 1985) to portfolio placement (Elbow & Belanoff, 1986) and now to student self-placement. The specific goals of placement systems can and should vary by local contexts, but Edward M. White and Cassie A. Wright (2016) provide a representative orientation: "a good placement system (somewhat of a rarity) is institutionally efficient because it arranges students in convenient teaching groups and is also valuable for

---

[8] I use the word "developers" to refer to those who work on DSP systems: teaching and non-teaching staff, tenured and non-tenure-track faculty, graduate and undergraduate students, and many others. I use this word to highlight the intense technical design role of those who contribute to the development and ongoing maintenance of DSP systems. I use "WPAs" when I wish to draw attention to disciplinary insights and/or more traditional WPA skills/labor. I make this distinction because if I am positioning students as *users* of DSP, it coheres to position WPAs as *developers* of those systems. I also find "developers" to be a more elegant and less hierarchical way to refer to the broad range of staff, students, and faculty who administer placement.

instructors because it gives them relatively homogenous groups to work with" (p. vi). This need for institutional efficiency often determines placement designs, and this orientation to placement as a homogenizing sorting mechanism is widely accepted across higher education. Blakesley (2003) summarizes the issue well: "The status quo has been that the institution should make decisions for the students, even when students might be better served to make those decisions themselves" (p. 37). But as Blakesley (2003) and others argue, DSP can offer challenges to this orientation on both theoretical and practical levels.

Within the realm of writing placement/assessment, DSP scholarship has a strong history of attending to student agency and power relations (Balay & Nelson, 2012; Kenner, 2016; Moos & Van Zanen, 2019; Royer & Gilles, 1998), suggesting that DSP bolsters student self-efficacy, institutional knowledge and awareness, and student *and* teacher satisfaction with courses; validity and reliability (Gere et al., 2010; Gere et al., 2013; Toth & Aull, 2014), providing evidence that well-designed DSP systems are effective placement/assessment tools; and design, purposes, and practicalities (Aull, 2021; Jones, 2008; Royer & Gilles, 2003, 2012), which has helped foster more localized implementations. On the whole, these studies demonstrate that DSP models have much to offer writing programs in terms of local adaptability, administrator usability and feasibility, and student agency (Saenkhum, 2016). Since its introduction to writing studies with Royer & Gilles' "Directed Self-Placement: An Attitude of Orientation" in *College Composition and Communication* in 1998, DSP has been a bedrock for writing placement innovation. But DSP has also been enlightened and encumbered by many well-intentioned concerns (Bedore & Rossen-Knill, 2004; Condon et al., 2001; Isaacs & Keohane, 2012; Neal & Huot, 2003; Nicolay, 2002; Schendel & O'Neill, 1999; Sullivan, 2008; Sullivan & Nielsen, 2009). Some arguments include:

1. Administrators evading responsibilities, I.E. requiring students to do evaluative labor that should be done by administrators (Condon et al., 2001, p. 204);

2. Administrators forcing students to participate in their own surveillance and subordination, I.E. to essentially "report back" to administrators their internalized oppression, biases, and trauma (Schendel & O'Neill, 1999, p. 200);

3. Lack of rigorous assessment validation, particularly in terms of consequential validity—both for students and for faculty, administrators, and staff (Harrington, 2005; Neal & Huot, 2003; Schendel & O'Neill, 1999);

4. The traditional placement systems that DSP seeks to replace are not *inherently* ineffectual (Neal & Huot, 2003); and

5. Student ignorance or inability to select appropriate courses, including lack of disciplinary expertise (Nicolay, 2002) and overall preparedness (Isaacs & Keohane, 2012).

These concerns were not taken lightly, and they demonstrate the breadth of intricate issues at work in writing placement. This scholarly ambivalence resulted in decades of validation efforts by scholars such as Anne Ruggles Gere, Mya Poe, Asao B. Inoue, Christie Toth, and Laura Aull. The work of these and many other scholars has enabled WPAs across the U.S. to make rhetorically sound, well-researched arguments about the value, efficiency, and usefulness of such placement methods for writing programs. Without these in-depth theorization and validation efforts, DSP might not be a viable placement option for WPAs today. Additionally, there has been a sizeable amount of validation and scholarship regarding DSP for multilingual students (Crusan, 2006, 2011; Das Bender, 2011; Ferris et al., 2017; Ferris & Lombardi, 2020; Saenkhum, 2016), which has largely been concerned with student agency, equity, and the arguably more complex context of multilingual student placement (including, but not limited to, institutional policies regarding language proficiency exams, academic advising, and international transfer articulation). These studies demonstrate not only DSP's ability to be both flexible and scalable, but also its usefulness across diverse student populations.

DSP initiated from (1) a lack of satisfaction with traditional placement systems like essay/portfolio scoring and sorting by exam scores, including teacher and student frustrations, and (2) the lack of statistical reliability of these other methods (the statistician working with Royer & Gilles famously said that the placement statistics were so random that they "might just as well let the students place themselves"; see Royer & Gilles, 1998, p. 60). In recent years, these concerns have been substantiated by research revealing standardized testing, such as the ACT and SAT, has predictive validity issues and largely measures wealth and race (Aguinis et al., 2016; Dixon-Román et al., 2013; Mattern et al., 2016). Notably for antiracist assessment, DSP has been shown to interrupt structural racism in placement systems by shifting demographic distributions of students in first-year composition courses to be more representative of the overall student population (Inoue, 2009a; Klausman & Lynch, 2022). This redistribution property of DSP has proven true at my institution as well. In looking at ten years of placement data at the University of Arizona, the results are promising: historically under-served student populations are now enrolling in *all* our first-year writing courses, not just our studio course, at percentages that more closely match their university student percentage. This shift happened slightly in our stop-gap year when we were implementing GPA-based placements and then became even more prominent when we shifted to DSP. Klausman and Lynch (2022) have recently found similar evidence in their community college context, reporting decreased enrollment in their developmental courses, which have been shown to have the opposite of their intended effect. In reporting on their switch from ACCUPLACER to "informed" self-placement (ISP), they state,

"As mentioned above, our ISP process has had a great benefit for incoming students of all races and ethnicities, as well as students with disabilities, low-income students, and other demographics. … Success rates have actually risen to 80 percent and continue to rise as faculty have embraced equity-minded pedagogical practices" (p. 78). By disaggregating their data not just by race but also by other demographic factors, such as disability and Pell Grant recipients, Klausman and Lynch (2022) show how DSP has the potential to disrupt not just systemic racism but also system ableism and classism. Despite its complexities, the data shows that DSP can be an effective and equitable placement assessment.

Christie Toth (2018) (she/her pronouns) usefully summarizes these efforts as "validation for social justice" (p. 145), suggesting that DSP in particular could be well-suited for strengthening placement equity as long as there are validation efforts at the local level. There has also been increasing interest in DSP for two-year colleges (Gilman et al., 2019; Klausman et al., 2016; Toth, 2018, 2019), which tend to serve more diverse student populations than their four-year university counterparts and are vital pathways to higher education. As evidenced by the recently published edited collection *Writing Placement in Two-Year Colleges: The Pursuit of Equity in Postsecondary Education* (Nastal et al., 2022) and the breadth of self-placement scholarship provided within, there is significant interest in DSP as a placement system for increasing equity and opportunities for student success. When analyzing DSP's potential to serve community college populations, Toth (2018) writes, "DSP's ability to achieve that promise [of social justice] is contingent on processes designed with a critical awareness of ideologies that reproduce social inequalities. … This labor must be undertaken carefully, critically, and continuously" (p. 151). When situated within the Fourth Wave of writing assessment scholarship

(Behm & Miller, 2012), DSP must be understood as a social justice endeavor, especially because placement has serious implications for student success.

An Advocacy Model of DSP

In addition to being a site of social justice, DSP is also a highly intercultural and technical communicative system. DSP can be validated not just by construct validity (I.E. composition studies content) or consequential validity frameworks (I.E. grades, course distribution, DFW—drop, fail, withdrawal—rates, retention, etc.) but also by the social justice and design standards of TPC method/ologies. Within a participatory localization and disability justice framework, I position DSP as advocacy, thus answering Poe et al.'s (2018) call to realize how "writing assessment best serves students when justice is taken as the ultimate aim of assessment" (p. 5). By centering student empowerment as its ultimate goal, DSP systems can accomplish their goal of equitable means of placement.

It must be said that placement is an incredibly complex site of academic institutional policy, articulation agreements, state mandates, and national education standards (particularly with common college examinations). Local placement systems must consider an intricately tangled web of policy, curricula, and course credit articulation across international, national, state, local, institutional, and programmatic levels. What's important about this tangled web is that DSP doesn't always interrupt these systems, but it does force developers to make its consequences explicit. Additionally, unlike placement systems in which students submit written work and wait for their placement, or in which student examination scores and high-school GPAs are used to sort and rank them, DSP systems begin with the assumption of dialogue and of student choice. The responsibility of developers in this dialogic system is to provide students with sufficient information to make an informed choice. As Toth (2019) so helpfully puts it, "The twin fundamentals of DSP are thus *guidance* and *choice*." Because of the weight placed on the guidance portion of the DSP equation, developers take great pains to ensure comprehensive information and instructions. The relevant program- and course-level outcomes (and their contexts, purposes, and values) are not always easy to explain, particularly to those outside of writing studies, and most of the transfer/articulation policies impacting their choices aren't simple, either, especially for international and transfer students.

It is this vital need to explain expert information to non-experts where I begin positioning DSP as technical communication. According to the Society for Technical Communication (n.d., 2015), the characteristics of technical communication are as follows:

1. Communicating about technical or specialized topics, such as computer applications, medical procedures, or environmental regulations;

2. Communicating by using technology, such as web pages or social media sites; and

3. Providing instructions about how to do something, regardless of how technical the task is or even if technology is used to create or distribute that communication.

Like many instructional materials, DSP corresponds well to these definitions. First, one of the key components of DSP is *guidance*. In a DSP system, developers must communicate some, if not all, of the following items:

- First-year writing curriculum, I.E. the courses available, their differences, and their sometimes complex sequences;

- Any additional curriculum options, I.E. transfer student courses, advanced composition, writing emphasis courses in the major, etc.;

- How these course/sequences satisfy (or *don't*—this information in particular should be transparent) academic program and graduation requirements;

- Individual course goals/outcomes (and thus program outcomes);

- The ways in which students' unique histories and contexts can impact the available choices, if at all (I.E. being able to "skip" the first course in a sequence through examination scores, dual enrollment, or other transfer credits, in accordance with institutional policy and state articulation agreements);

- Which student behaviors, skills, learning preferences, and academic/interpersonal needs are best suited for the available choices (and why);

- How to complete the placement process, including potentially completing a digital questionnaire and/or writing task, submitting relevant documentation to appropriate parties in particular document formats, selecting a course, and/or communicating with relevant advisory bodies; and

- If appropriate for the local context, examples of course activities, assignments, assessments, sample student writing, and/or syllabi.

Weaving all these various nodes of vital information into the DSP system takes considerable time and effort. It also requires technical writing: a strong enough understanding of the complex systems to communicate the most relevant information succinctly *and* comprehensively, and especially in plain, widely accessible language rather than disciplinary jargon. While some students may be familiar with such terminology, presuming universal student (and parent) familiarity with specialized terminology enacts some of the harmful systemic and pedagogical racism illuminated by scholars like April Baker-Bell (2013) and many others (see Inoue, 2015; Ketai, 2012; Kynard, 2013; Lyiscott, 2018). In this vein, DSP developers must make their specialized knowledge not just cogent and well-organized but also *usable*. For DSP to achieve its purpose of empowerment, students must be able to apply this information if they are to decide which course best meets their goals and needs.

Second, writing itself is a technology (Brooke & Grabill, 2016), and so are assessments (Huot, 2002; Scott & Inoue, 2016), and DSP is now largely mediated through multiple technologies/modalities. While many students will be familiar with online surveys and questionnaires, we cannot make assumptions about students' levels of technological access, skills, or ability. Nor do all DSP systems use questionnaires; some use primarily in-person advising and/or group orientations, while some use a mixture of digital and analogue methods (Toth, 2019). And because DSP systems often ask students to interact with other media to access the entire system, including things like hyperlinks, videos, and supplemental text documents, this aspect of DSP (as mediated through technology) is doubly important. In design and iteration phases of any student-facing system, especially one as vital as placement, student insights about accessibility and usability is crucial.

Finally, providing usable instructions for completing the DSP and selecting a course is the crux of any student self-placement system. While DSP developers must determine which crucial details to include, they must also provide instructions for questionnaire completion, course selection, and other processes (including clicking on the all-important "submit" button). Equally important is the way in which the *choice*, the second fundamental of DSP, is articulated to the students. Most campuses have a placement culture of examination and ranking. On my campus, for example, Foundations Writing is the only unit that implements a student self-placement system; the other two Foundations units, Mathematics and Foreign Language, both use proficiency exams to place students. Students thus often encounter DSP as an outlier, and even when instructions are clear and explicit, uptake is not guaranteed. In addition to instructions for managing the DSP tool, this ideological shift in orientation to student self-placement must also be communicated to students in accessible and usable ways.

While this three-pronged definition from the Society for Technical Communication (n.d.) provides an overview of technical communication from industry standards, I also find salience in positioning DSP as advocacy. Natasha N. Jones' (2016) overview of social justice orientations to and methodologies for TPC align well with disability justice principles. Jones argues that critical approaches to equity and social justice can help legitimate TPC by more precisely addressing the ways in which communication and technology mediate the human experience, including that of those who are historically and contemporarily oppressed (2016, p. 343). Arguing for a humanistic understanding of TPC, Jones writes, "Oppression then is central to the definition of social justice in TPC because understanding that oppression must be addressed collectively by enhancing and supporting the agency of others is foundationally humanistic" (p. 348). This shift toward the inclusion of social justice concerns in disciplinary conversations is certainly not new. For example, Frey et al. (1996) suggest ways communication studies can benefit from including systematic approaches to social justice and equity. They usefully outline a "social justice sensibility" that includes four features. This sensibility:

1. Foregrounds ethical concerns;

2. Commits to structural analyses of ethical problems;

3. Adopts an activist orientation; and

4. Seeks identification with others. (p. 111)

By calling for an "activist orientation" (p. 111), they remind readers that social justice requires *action*: not just the illumination of inequities but also movement toward addressing and redressing them. By calling for "identification with others," they highlight the importance of solidarity, not as charity or kindness, but as what some call allyship (Del Hierro et al., 2016; Wible, 2019). Some offer the term "accomplice" as a critical reframing of "ally" (Powell & Kelly, 2017), providing means for allies to critically reflect on positionalities, goals, values, biases, and actions. Though these social justice concerns are not new, they are becoming more important as our sociopolitical context shifts and as academic institutions, units, and programs continue adding diversity and equity outcomes to their programmatic goals and mission statements. This particular historical moment calls for such work, and there must be substantive activist-oriented models of fairness for WPAs.

I suggest that, like all assessment tools, DSP can be—but isn't automatically—a form of advocacy. As teachers and as administrators, we hold a powerful positionality: in some ways, we exist between students and the institution, and we can mediate certain aspects of their interactions. Historically in composition studies, we have done our best to mitigate and dissolve power imbalances, but there remains a hierarchy wherein undergraduate students are positioned as those least informed and least qualified to intervene in their own education. For me as an educator and administrator, this intangible space between students and the institution feels often like translation (providing students with more usable versions of unparsable institutional discourse and practices) and often like a trail guide (showing students alternate pathways, signs of trouble, and how and when to access help). Assessment and placement also exists in this space, as it communicates between the student and the institution, often in shorthand. This is a space in which advocacy is crucial. I suggest positioning DSP as advocacy because it seeks to make placement an accessible, comprehensive, empowering, and unambiguous process, and because it seeks to actively intervene in structural academic marginalization and oppression. For students, DSP can reframe placement as a process in which their input is valued and in fact prioritized, which is ultimately an act of resistance against that hierarchical structure upheld by the institution. Truly trusting students can be revolutionary, but providing guidance on what that means is also necessary. DSP does this already, which is why user-driven and participatory methodologies are so important to its design, implementation, and iteration: it lets developers focus on the humanness of the process and product.

As this overview demonstrates, DSP is a highly complex social action involving many stakeholders, systems, technologies, and objectives. Communicating pertinent details effectively requires significant downshifting and technical maneuvering. Because DSP seeks to make much of our field's specialized knowledge usable, I submit that participatory localization and UX method/ologies are highly relevant to the design, implementation, and revision of DSP processes. Especially when positioning TPC as advocacy work (Jones, 2016). This lens can thus help us understand DSP better by orienting us to conceptions of communities that include students as users. In particular, the participatory aspect of these method/ologies is fundamental not only to DSP but any equity- or justice-oriented assessment project.

Aligning Localization Theories for DSP

A crucial component of any writing assessment practice is localization. Broadly articulated, localization is a type of contextualization, a means of attuning to the local and communal. Localization is also both reflective and reflexive, and it provides an orientation to writing assessment that diverges from those found in other disciplines, asking developers to withhold demands for efficiency and standardization and instead focus on the specific context of the evaluation situation they seek to develop. Drawing on the work of Pamela Moss (1994a,

1994b, 1998) and others, Huot (2002) articulates a cohesive set of principles for localization for writing studies, stating that assessments ought to be: (1) site based; (2) locally controlled; (3) context sensitive; (4) rhetorically based; and (5) accessible (p. 105). In the years since this initial work, these five principles have been cited as a foundation of localization in writing assessment. Huot later refined his understanding in collaboration with other scholars (O'Neill et al., 2009), adding that assessment should also be "theoretically consistent" (p. 57)—meaning it should remain consistent with its own local goals, values, implementation as well as with disciplinary best practices. Because of its role in assuring that assessments are relevant to and reflective of their local contexts, localization is necessary for successful feedback loops, which are a fundamental aspect of writing assessment (Schendel & Macauley, 2012). Writing placement especially has been noted as a site requiring intensive localization (Adler-Kassner & O'Neill, 2010), mostly because of the intricate conflux of stakeholders, policies, and goals I outline above. Those details change drastically by site, leading many assessment scholars to understand that an assessment that serves one unit or population may not necessarily serve another. For this reason, the development of a placement tool/system must include some aspect of localization.

In TPC, localization has a different set of connotations, purposes, and methods from traditional writing assessment scholarship, instead aiming at contextualizing for the purpose of improving the developers' understandings of the target user group and thus the tool/technology in its context(s). Shivers-McNair and San Diego (2017) find in their collaborative work four dimensions of cross-cultural localization: (1) localizing community; (2) localizing goals; (3) localizing communication; and (4) localizing inclusion. These dimensions provide more precise ways to prioritize and implement DSP as localized advocacy: rather than operating under pre-set, outdated, or rigid assumptions of student needs, creating dialogues that work toward defining and achieving shared goals. Through modeling these collaborative localization practices, Shivers-McNair and San Diego (2017) argue that words such as *user*, *community*, and *diversity* must also be situated locally and be responsive to ever-shifting contexts. For WPAs, this practice could translate to critically and recursively considering how *students* are defined at their institution and in their program. Additionally, Sun (2012) provides a useful distinction between developer localization and user localization, with the latter differentiated by their users' experience "incorporating the technology into one's life" (p. 40). In the DSP context, *developer* localization often includes the traditional assessment localization of program outcomes and their related constructs (WPA concerns), whereas *user* localization focuses on the user perspective and experience: usability, accessibility, user interface, offered pathways, and more (student concerns). Tanita Saenkhum (2016) reminds us of how many complex interlocking factors play a role in student self-placement, and though we cannot predict all the possible factors, UX can help prevent weak localization, mitigate irrelevant, outdated, and/or racist/ableist construct representations, and prevent inaccessible designs.[9] Below, I describe three examples—three stories—of my local institution, demonstrating the various ways (large and small) that UX can help localize placement assessment as well as promote more theoretically sound, accessible, and equitable DSP design.

Stories of Localizing through UX

The full implementation of a DSP system for the University of Arizona (UArizona) Foundations Writing Program (WP) has been ongoing for many years, but the initial design for a

---

[9] "Construct representation" is the assessment theory phrase for assessment items that match their conceptual definition, such as what a local writing program defines as "writing" and how that manifests in the assessment. See Chapter 2 for a more thorough discussion.

DSP tool began in 2014. By 2016, when CollegeBoard made changes to their SAT scoring procedures, UArizona WPAs were ready to shift from an algorithm-based placement to a self-placement system. This kairotic moment offered many institutions across the country, including ours, an opportunity to explore other placement systems, but the shift didn't occur overnight: developing any digital DSP system is always complicated, and even more so for incoming cohorts of over 10,000 students. By the launch in 2018, the DSP system at UArizona came to be known as the Foundations Writing Evaluation (FWE), with two distinct off-shoots including the international FWE (iFWE) and online FWE (oFWE), each of which incorporate some aspects of the original FWE. It's hosted by Qualtrics and monitored perennially by a dedicated twelve-month administrative staff member and a rotating band of graduate assistant administrators and placement advisors. These various FWE systems are intricate and not simple to maintain, especially during peak orientation and enrollment seasons. For us, UX was a much-needed intervention because of the demands on our one full-time placement WPA to develop (and maintain) multiple FWEs across different campuses and student populations. This internal exigence was exciting in that it demonstrated institutional buy-in and desirable implications for more efficient enrollment management, but the demand also meant increased labor and, along with it, increased chances of weak localization across the FWE variations.

The FWE system at the UArizona currently has several features, among them: (1) a Qualtrics online survey tool; (2) year-round asynchronous email advising; (3) synchronous orientation session advising; and (4) a "Handy Guide to Foundations Writing" webpage. We currently have a different Qualtrics tool for different student populations: international students, main campus students, Global Direct students (international online campus), and AZ Online campus students. The Qualtrics tool is the central feature of the DSP process, and it relies on an internal web service that reads secure student information (such as transcripts) that can, while the student takes the FWE, filter relevant information regarding their course/sequence options. The Qualtrics tool also implements a self-assessment questionnaire that inquires about student histories with various literacy tasks and learning preferences. Through this survey, students can report pending dual enrollment/transfer credits as well as relevant exam scores, can select a course, and can request additional support from placement advisors. Most of the FWEs include a course recommendation, a writing task (or two), and a link to the Handy Guide, which offers descriptions of the courses, sample assignment guides, and sample class activities.

In the following sections, I present three method/ologies for DSP: (1) UX design research; (2) usability studies; and (3) embedded reflective opportunities. These sections each describe potential methods of utilizing student input and seeking collaboration on the design, implementation, and iteration of a DSP. These method/ologies demonstrate both small-scale and large-scale ways of enacting participatory localization.

UX Design Research

As I've noted, placement assessment is incredibly messy. Thankfully, UX helps reduce some of the messiness, at least on the students' side: the easier the process, the more likely students are to matriculate, enroll, and persist through their programs. For WPAs, UX offers solutions to questions of equity, accessibility, user-friendliness, uptake, and localization. UX methods can be shaped to address any of these concerns. In terms of overarching frameworks, UX prioritizes the user's lived experience and honors the user's knowledge. The Nielsen Norman Group, an industry leader in UX research, supports an empathy- and advocacy-based approach to UX. They write, "As UX professionals, it is our job to advocate on behalf of the user" (Gibbons,

2018). Other industry models have similar priorities. The Creative Reaction Lab (n.d.) offers

their approach, called *Equity-Centered Community Design*, which prioritizes empathy,

collaborative creation, engagement with the communities in which/with whom they work, and an

approach to power, which must be "acknowledged, dismantled, and/or shared." Likewise, the

Design Justice Network (2018) advocates for similar principles that align well with disability

justice and other coalitional approaches to UX and design. In these models, the communities

determine the methods used. Some UX methods include: diary studies, journey mapping,

prototype testing, empathy mapping, and task analyses. The feasibility and adaptability of these

methods across contexts is one of their strengths, and part of the localization process for DSP is

to determine (iteratively and collaboratively) which UX frameworks and methods best align with

the community's needs.

At UArizona, over the course of 2021 and 2022, our developers requested IRB approval

and received funding to implement a student-focused UX/participatory design research study. In

particular, we were looking to revise our co-curricular courses, which would go on to help us

iterate on our course designs and curricula as well as our oFWE (the DSP serving specifically

our online campus students). In summer 2021, I conducted focus groups with students who had

completed ENGL197B, a co-curricular with our online ENGL101 & ENGL102 courses. A

published description of the results of the focus groups, as well as the subsequent coding and

analysis, are forthcoming (Kryger & Mitchum, 2023). To summarize, having conversations with

students about their experiences with the course and co-curricular provided surprising insights

into how to better localize our online campus course placements. We were not anticipating a

strong presence of transfer students in our focus groups, but we learned so much about their

unique challenges for transfer and placement: there are far fewer support structures for transfer students, especially adult returning students and distance/online students. Their concerns and issues allowed us to revise our DSP and corresponding curriculum with more precision and awareness. These focus groups are currently being followed up with other UX methods, such as usability testing of the new DSP questionnaire items, additional focus groups, and surveys about the co-curricular course modifications. Overall, UX is primed to help WPAs better serve students in accessible, contextual, recursive, and equitable ways by providing methodological frameworks and toolkits for student-centered and user-developed placement systems.

Usability Studies

As Miller-Cochran and Rodrigo (2009) so succinctly put it, "usability is about users" (p. 1). Usability testing, or usability studies, are intended to support the design process of any given technology. Perhaps as it implies, usability is generally understood to be about ease of use and usefulness, centering the needs and experiences of the users rather than the system's aesthetic or design. Some usability principles include learnability, readability, memorability, efficiency, error recovery, and satisfaction (Acharya, 2019).

For our DSP at UArizona, our developers conducted a usability study in Fall 2019 on the main campus FWE. For this usability study, they asked a group of university students to take the FWE and use Zoom to record their screen during the process. The students also participated in a follow-up large group discussion and a brief explanation of the process prior to testing. The results of the testing primarily revealed issues around user interface, content, sequences, and visuals. The developers wanted to know more about how students reacted to the questionnaire questions and the sequencing of DSP items such as the questionnaire, writing task, and follow-up questions. There were also broad ranges of affective responses to the FWE, particularly regarding the course recommendation, which is calculated based on the responses to the 19-item self-assessment questionnaire. We also learned that students were not accessing the supplemental materials. The results of the usability testing confirmed students didn't recognize that they had the power to choose a course for themselves. This data was used to think more carefully about the placement of information not just embedded within the FWE itself but also across other platforms where students gather information: namely the digital orientation platform used to deliver university requirements and orientation content to new students prior to their first semester and the Foundations Writing Program and FWE home webpages. For more details about the issues, goals, methods, results, and modifications, see the UX Portfolio of Aly Higgins (n.d.), one of the primary developers at the time.

This particular instance of implementing usability methods toward the improvement of an already existing DSP system was successful in that our team gathered useful data for iterating on the FWE, but the process was not without challenges or data limitations. For example, the users who participated in the usability study were user-adjacent to our target population, rather than users from our target population. They were not incoming students matriculating into the university, they were students who had already taken at least a semester of courses at UArizona, and they were largely late-career students. This positionality was further complicated because the majority of the students were also English majors with strong writing behaviors/skills. There also could have been a broader representation of students from different disciplines and educational backgrounds. Despite these study limitations, the results of the usability testing did contribute to revisions to the FWE before it went live in spring 2020 for the next wave of incoming students. In particular, we were able to revise the section sequencing, some of the inclusion of visuals/gifs, and more. The process of gathering student feedback on the usability of the FWE created opportunities to discuss both specific details of our DSP tool as well as broader concerns, such as the complications of transfer students completing the same self-assessment questionnaire items as the incoming first-year students.

Embedded Opportunities for Reflection

One unique facet of the UArizona FWE system is that the developers built into the design of the Qualtrics survey some mechanisms for collecting student feedback. We have thus been collecting data about student experiences with our DSP system since 2018. There are two primary sources of this phenomenological data: (1) optional, end-of-survey questionnaire items and (2) student responses to the reflection activity. Both have been useful to our developers and useful for gauging students' overall impressions of the process. The optional post-questionnaire items provide both qualitative and quantitative data. They are:

1. ITEM 1: "How useful did you find each of the following sections in helping you choose your writing course?" (5-point Likert scale per item listed)

    a. "Prior reading and writing experience"

    b. "Writing task"

    c. "Compare your writing with student samples"

    d. "Course recommendation"

    e. "Course descriptions"

2. ITEM 2: "What did you like and/or dislike about the Directed Self-Placement?" (open-ended question)

(Table 1)

These questions are sequenced at the end of the FWE, after the self-assessment, the writing task, and the course selection. The questions have no bearing on students' course selection and there's absolutely no obligation for students to respond. (Note that the FWE has since been revised, and the sections listed in Table 1 have been likewise revised.) Regardless, we have been able to use this data not only to revise design choices but also to update the section sequencing. These "feedback loop" items embedded into the FWE have been useful for our developers, but there are also methodological limitations for potentially validating or generalizing the data. For instance, our team has only been able to code a small number of the qualitative data, in part because of time/labor constraints and in part because of the sheer quantity of responses. It's also possible that the phrasing of the questions could have primed students, and the open-ended questions were often short and provided limited detail (Gevers & Whittig, 2019). When Gevers and Whittig presented these findings at CWPA in 2019, the placement team (including myself) were already brainstorming future methods of collecting student input. A few possible directions included: interviews and simulated recall with students, disparate impact analyses, and interviews with instructors (Gevers & Whittig, 2019).

The second and more recent source of data has been the implementation of a reflective writing task. Initially, the main FWE writing task asked students to read and respond to a brief article about the ethics of plagiarism, but in spring 2020, we switched the writing task to a reflective essay. This reflection task serves the following functions:

1. Provides students with an opportunity to practice reflective writing, such as reflecting on the self-assessment questionnaire and articulating which course best suits their needs

based on the evidence they've gathered (this item is a localization by our developers, as our curriculum heavily emphasizes reflection);

2. Provides developers with descriptive insights into student experiences with the various features of the FWE, the overall process, and our curriculum; and

3. Provides developers with aggregate areas of student experiences for future studies.

These embedded opportunities for reflection demonstrate how prompts for student feedback can be incorporated into the design of the DSP without having to develop separate studies.

Conclusion

The stories told here, and the labor, research, and conversations around them, are still ongoing. The Foundations Writing Program at UArizona is iteratively improving their online course curriculum based on the focus group data; we are continuing to rely on usability studies to determine factors relating to accessibility, engagement, and empowerment; and we are still collecting and reviewing data from the embedded reflection task and the optional reflection questions. But the conversations engendering these design decisions perhaps matter more: while the tools used are vital, and the ways in which they are designed have reverberating consequences, the justice-oriented frameworks of the developers have further-reaching impacts. We know these systems (as well as our students and communities) are always changing, and WPAs must be ever vigilant in designing for equity. For DSP, that means starting with placement's key stakeholders—students. As demonstrated above, UX and participatory localization method/ologies have incredible use value developers administering placement. Designing a student self-placement system is never easy, but including students in the process can bolster DSP localization efforts. User and usability localization are key components of TPC models, and content/construct localization has long been the priority for writing assessment; together, these approaches model a richer approach to localization that specifically attunes to students, their communities, and their needs. And finally, I frame DSP as advocacy because it seeks to actively intervene in structurally marginalizing placements. UX and participatory localization method/ologies can help us better achieve those dialogic goals and make writing placement assessment less a pain and more a pleasure.

Chapter Four

DEPATHOLOGIZING THE WRITING CLASSROOM

Neuronormativity is present everywhere. From the way temporality is constructed in educational settings, to the frequency with which my anxiety is treated as a vexing blight to cleanse from my psyche, neurological norms are ubiquitous. Norms of cognition and emotion are especially prevalent wherever reading and writing are used as a means of communication, knowledge-making, and the evaluation of learning. Writing is demanding on one's executive functioning and memory/recall (Kellogg & Raulerson, 2007), as well as emotion regulation (Eckert et al., 2016; Steel & Klingsieck, 2016). Students' abilities to read, write, edit, revise, research, reflect, and think are constructed alongside commonly accepted ideas of normate minds and bodies. Most of my time in educational settings has been occupied by learning how to mask and pass for neurotypical. I found ways to work around my challenges with mental "processing speed," emotion regulation, time blindness, and inattention—and these work-arounds, even bolstered by standard studying practices, require so much additional time and energy. Most of my "neurotic" coping mechanisms were the result of my anxiety about not doing well in school and about being seen as stupid, slow, lazy, or "ditzy."

Neuronormativity is conceptually akin to Sami Schalk's (2018) discussion of *able-mindedness*, which she argues is "the socially constructed norm of mental capacity and ability that is typically posed in binary opposition to mental disability" (p. 61). These norms are what sustain stigmatizing language of mental ability. They also sustain well-intentioned but harmful pedagogical practices through a culture of punishment, control, and surveillance in the classroom. For Schalk, able-mindedness includes concepts like "rationality, reasonableness, sanity, intelligence, mental agility, self-awareness, social awareness, and control of thoughts and behaviors" (p. 61). Mental agility, for example, contributes to information recall and processing, which supports students' ability to respond quickly and cogently when called on in class; measurements of intelligence, for example, are historically racially discriminatory and yet still form many of the foundations of not just academic endeavors, but also mental diagnoses (Metzl, 2010). Normative assumptions about things like intelligence, rationality, and sanity permeate educational settings in ways that remain largely natural, neutral, and tacit. In *Mad at School: Rhetorics of Mental Disability and Academic Life* (2011), Margaret Price identifies eleven topoi of academia that constitute her understanding of neuronormativity: "rationality, criticality, presence, participation, resistance, productivity, collegiality, security, coherence, truth, and independence" (p. 5). Just like Schalk's able-mindedness concepts, commonplaces such as coherence, collegiality, and rationality are assumed inherent in all students, and there are consequences for being found lacking. How many of these concepts are requisite for "good" writing, for "effective" communication? In what ways do writing instructors discuss, teach, grade, and/or penalize the absence of these concepts? How are students instructed to assess their own communicative abilities, if not through these concepts? How can we support writing classrooms that enable non-normative ways of thinking, learning, and being?

Neuronormativity is the package of socially constructed rules that substantiate and maintain the pathology paradigm—the set of ableist ideologies governing such norms. The neurodiversity paradigm, Walker's (2021) answer to the pathology paradigm, provides a set of more open, inclusive, and flexible ideologies. In the neurodiversity paradigm, neuroqueering can create resistance against the delimiting norms of the pathology paradigm. For Walker (2021) and Yergeau (2018), neurodivergence and queerness are deeply interconnected. 'Neuroqueer' is the word they use to signal the counteracting of both neuronormativity and cishetero/allonormativity. In writing classrooms, neuroqueering can take many shapes, but practices and policies around grading are particularly thorny areas full of opportunities to explore structural neuronormativity and ways in which teachers may (de) and (re)construct it. Ultimately, when writing assessment practices are flexible rather than fixed, they can help teachers resist normative expectations of control and dominance over their students.

Despite being an invention of the twentieth century, grading has become so pervasive it seems inevitable. But grading is neither value-neutral nor apolitical, and it's certainly not inevitable. Grading as we know it comes from a long history of twentieth-century behaviorism, the rise of industrialization and efficiency/productivity, and the use of schools as social sorting mechanisms (Feldman, 2019). These and other factors contribute to a modern misrepresentation of grading as an objective and neutral means of assessment. Despite functioning as institutional and social ranking/sorting mechanisms, grades are not accurate representations of student learning (Elbow, 1994; Kohn, 2006, 2012). Though grades are precious commodities (rife with social, financial, and affective consequences) exchanged for good behavior and meeting teacher expectations, they're also inconsistent and subjective. Grades are, as students and teachers know all too well, incommensurable: even when given a common rubric, raters are never fully consistent (Stevenson, 2019). Elbow (1994) writes, "In short, the reliability in holistic scoring is not a measure of how texts are valued by real readers in natural settings, but only of how they are valued in artificial settings with imposed agreements" (p. 189). Even such imposed agreements are rarely consistent. Based on its function as a selective mechanism, grading also focuses on control, discipline, and ranking. These foci are, as teacher-scholars such as Elbow (1994), Blum (2020), Kohn (2012), and Carillo (2021) note, the antithesis of learning. Whether well-intentioned or not, grades actually communicate very little about actual learning (Huot, 2002) and can even have the opposite effect on students. Research shows that grades function socially and affectively (Inman & Powell, 2018), often spurring aversive emotions and distracting students from learning (Kohn, 2012). All told, our cultural fixation on grades is annoying at best and detrimental at worst: they actively interrupt student learning. Teachers of all levels and disciplines can benefit from rethinking how neuronormativity is structured in our classrooms, especially through assessment.

Because of its roles of ranking and sorting, writing assessments are sites of social justice (Behm & Miller, 2012). They are socially constructed technologies that do not escape bias and inequitable structures of power and privilege (Inoue, 2015). For these reasons, grading practices must address and disrupt systemic oppression. Because writing assessments are socio-politically mediated technologies that function within larger systems of power and privilege (Inoue, 2009b), grading practices are also sites of "structural violence" (Lederman & Warwick, 2018) and trauma (Stommel, 2021a). As such, White supremacy functions within our classrooms and in particular our language standards (see Inoue, 2019). White supremacy works alongside systems of imperialism, patriarchy, capitalism, and ableism, and these systems inform and support each other (Piepzna-Samarasinha, 2018). Lederman and Warwick (2018) argue that to address the structural violence inherent in writing assessment systems, assessments must be designed with that purpose in mind: with justice at the forefront, not as an add-on (also known as a *retrofit*; see Dolmage, 2017) later in the course or assignment design process.

Neuronormativity is constantly being constructed and (re)inforced in academic institutions, and it's reified in so much of writing assessment. This chapter takes a critical look at a few loci of neuronormative assumptions and policing (often through grading) in writing classrooms. In the first section, Laziness and Procrastination, I examine the ways in which assessment is attuned to student labor and pathologizes laziness, as well as how a cultural obsession with productivity comes alive in harrowing ways in colleges and universities. In the second section, Time and Control, I demonstrate how neuronormative assumptions and obsessions with time disadvantage neurodivergent students, and I situate these norms within a need for controlling and surveilling student behavior and production. In the third section, Trust and Disclosure, I argue for the importance of fundamentally trusting students and the importance of discussing disclosure. Finally, in the Implementation section, I provide some methods for disrupting the demands of neuronormativity placed on teachers.

Laziness & Procrastination

Laziness is a neuronormative, ableist myth. American cultural norms of labor, success, and independence have ableist implications and consequences. When productivity is tied to personhood, any disability that directly impacts one's labor ability or output is disparaged not as a social construct but as a personal failing. As Devon Price (they/them pronouns) explains in *Laziness Does Not Exist* (2021), "Our culture has us convinced that success requires nothing more than willpower, that pushing ourselves to the point of collapse is morally superior to taking it easy" (p. 15). While these cultural assumptions about hard work and laziness may seem harmless, they are deeply salient for disabled students, especially neurodivergent students. Depression, for example, is often reduced to merely laziness, often characterized as a weakness in personality or as a moral failure born of a fundamental lacking. Yet people with depression spend most of their body's energy in survival mode, which not only requires unseen effort but can also worsen one's ability to labor in conventional ways. Price (2021) summarizes their psychological research into a phenomenon they call The Laziness Lie, which they see as comprised of three key tenets: "1. Your worth is your productivity. 2. You cannot trust your own feelings and limits. 3. There is always more you could be doing" (p. 15). In classroom settings, these tenets and their byproducts produce a great deal of shame, anxiety, and fear, aversive emotions that make focus, motivation, and emotion regulation more difficult. Many students feel trapped by perfectionism, the fear of disappointing others and the fear of failing (though most composition scholars agree writing is imperfectible; see Inoue, 2014; Rose, 2016). So many of us try to meet standards that are amorphous, ill-defined, ever-shifting. To use a sports metaphor, the goal posts are always moving further and further away, urging us to work more and more, urging us to deny our bodyminds to fulfill our productivity-based role in a capitalist society. When combined with neurological differences that are quite unwelcome in educational settings, The Laziness Lie's impact on student learning can be devastating.

One of the most common ways The Laziness Lie infiltrates writing classrooms is through procrastination. The phenomenon of procrastination is so commonplace it's become part of the lore of college writing: unless externally motivated, most students will wait until the last minute to write a paper. Procrastination is often subsumed under the laziness category (I.E., I should always be working harder, working smarter, writing more, increasing efficiency, increasing laudable output). Process-oriented pedagogies (Beaufort, 2007; Crowley, 1998; Elbow, 1981) have limited some procrastination tendencies, as students are less likely to procrastinate the writing of an entire essay if the project is strategically parceled out for them and if those more frequent steps are lower-stakes than a single final term paper worth 30% of their course grade. But procrastination still happens even with process pedagogies. It just takes different forms, such as incomplete outlines/drafts or avoiding peer review for fear of negative feedback/having an incomplete draft. My own personal experiences as a student, tutor, and teacher reiterate this point. In my years as a writing center tutor, I saw many of these variations of procrastination and their effects: I saw the guilt, the stress, the internalized shame, the fear. I heard students' very logical and reasonable explanations, their fears of disclosing their issues or asking questions of their instructors. In working with these students, I wanted to find ways to avoid such things in my own classroom. As an undergraduate student, I had too much generalized anxiety to procrastinate for long (a benefit of that aspect of my neurodivergence, an affordance folks with depression or other divergences may not have) but as a tutor, I understood my peers' concerns. When I began teaching, I realized that process pedagogies alone are insufficient: they must be paired with other practices, and other values, if there is to be less procrastination and/or avoidance in writing classrooms. This is not to say that it is teachers' prerogative to manage or reduce students' emotional dysregulation; the goal is to instead structure our writing programs and classrooms so that we, as the 10 Principles of Disability Justice states, "leave no bodymind behind" (Sins Invalid, 2015, 2019).

Social and educational psychology research conducted on procrastination in the last two decades is illuminating. This body of research argues procrastination happens more frequently when the task matters to them (Deemer et al., 2014) and that fear of failure is a common precursor to procrastination, particularly in women (Özer et al., 2009). Studies also indicate procrastination is connected to the affective domain, suggesting procrastination is a "failure" of self-regulation (Eckert et al., 2016). Eckert and his colleagues investigate the ways in which emotion regulation impacts procrastination, which they define as "a dysfunctional response to undesired affective states" (p. 10). Drawing from the work of Berking et al. (2008, 2014) and Eckert et al. (2016), emotion regulation can be summarized as the following abilities:

- Awareness of one's emotions;

- Identifying and labeling one's emotions;

- Interpreting one's emotions (including their relation to bodily sensations);

- Understanding the prompts of one's emotions;

- Accepting one's emotions;

- Supporting oneself in distressing situations (self-support);

- Tolerating and/or confronting one's aversive emotions (resilience); and

- Modifying one's aversive emotions (modification).

While resilience and modification are considered by Eckert et al. (2016) and Berking et al. (2008) to be the two abilities that most modulate the others, many of them are related to procrastination. The inability to notice or identify one's emotional state, for example, can lead to task aversion: if I don't know I'm afraid of my teacher's feedback on my writing (and that it is potentially leading to avoidance), it's much easier to assume I'm lazy, stupid, or just a bad student than it is to address that fear or its source(s). If, then, the feedback and subsequent grades mirror these unspoken fears and internal shame-talk, the aversion digs its claws in that much deeper. Of course, such aversions manifest in many ways: I.E. students avoiding class, avoiding peer review days, avoiding reading a teacher's feedback, frequent procrastination (which is then further exacerbated by students' hectic lives and demanding schedules). Aversive emotions such as guilt and shame also worsen emotion regulation, making procrastination a difficult cycle to break, especially for those who experience difficulties (I.E. emotion "dysregulation") as an aspect of their non-normative minds.

Irregular mood and emotion-regulation challenges are also considered by the American Psychiatric Association's (2013) *Diagnostic and Statistical Manual of Mental Disorders* (5th ed.;

DSM-5) to be a comorbidity of ADHD: "Emotional dysregulation or emotional impulsivity commonly occurs in children and adults with ADHD. Individuals with ADHD self-report and are described by others as being quick to anger, easily frustrated, and overreactive emotionally (Barkley, 2015; Shaw et al., 2014; van Stralen, 2016)." I've struggled with emotion regulation for as long as I can remember, and it's always been dismissed (disparaged) as feminine hypersensitivity. I now know that I have chronic illnesses and neurodivergent traits that shape how my bodymind processes and deals with emotions. Even as an adult with intentionally developed emotional intelligence, modulating my emotions is still difficult. I often work hard enough to pass for neurotypical, to mask as "normal." I learned a long time ago to save my breakdowns for private spaces, like bathrooms on campus or the yoga mat at home. This effort toward masking, which enables me to present myself as a productive academic and valuable member of society, is exhausting. Those who are historically marginalized and/or non-normative must work extra hard to deal with racist, ableist, sexist, capitalist standards: there's the emotional labor of constantly managing others' expectations and warding off bigotry, but also the effort needed to pass, mask, or circumnavigate. This additional labor and emotional exhaustion then lives in the body, which we're enculturated to mistrust and mistreat. When success is correlated to hard work, mental and physical exhaustion is both valorized and compulsory.

The Laziness Lie underscores much of the neuronormativity embedded in assumptions about students and their academic performance. Simply put, punishing students for "laziness" (I.E. procrastination, late work, tardiness, lack of engagement, etc.) punishes neurodivergence. In this way, writing assessments measure students' neurological normativity, their proximity to normate, their ability to pass/mask as neurotypical, or even environmental factors, things over which students often have little or no control: their living space(s), access to reliable internet or other technology, work and school schedules, caretaking obligations, lack of access to proper care or sustenance. All these factors impact students' academic performance in class, and none of them accurately measure student learning.

Additionally, humans' attention spans are competing over more content, more demands on our time, and more ways to stay engaged than ever before. Some quick facts:

- "The volume of unique information the average person encounters in a day is approximately five times what the average person encountered in 1986";

- "According to IBM, 2.5 quintillion bytes of data are added every single day"; and

- "Ninety percent of the information currently available on the internet was added in the past two years." (Price, 2021, p. 137)

This exponential increase in unique information and the sheer amount of data now accessible to humans is staggering. When neurotypical students who have a so-called "normal" attention span or mental storage space struggle to manage so much data and information, what does that mean for students with non-normative attention spans and memory? If the "average" student is overwhelmed, what does that mean for students with proximity to anxiety and depression? Often "attention" is discussed as a bottomless well, an infinite resource to be accessed whenever necessary. Research shows that's wrong—people's attention spans can wax and wane, can shrink or expand, can be diminished by environmental factors and the intensity of demand. As Price (2021) helpfully explains, "Our attention is less like a laser beam (which can be pointed at any single specific point we desire) and more like a rotating lighthouse lantern, temporarily bathing individual rocks in light as it continues to spin across its surroundings" (p. 84). I find this orientation to "attention" instructive for many reasons, particularly because Price's research suggests that what has come to represent "normal" cognitive functioning, such as being able to sit through an entire class period or Zoom meeting without being distracted, isn't as typical as people believe. Price (2021) advises that creativity, problem solving, empathy, and even our ability to resist biased thinking are all improved when humans are allowed to take breaks and have adequate rest (p. 86). Price also suggests that behaviors that socially read as "laziness" are actually the body's way of protecting us from things like burnout and cognitive, physical, and/or emotional overload (p. 52). Especially for those of us who are disabled and neurodivergent, these protections often come at the cost of social capital, passing or masking, professional advancement, and more. The research shows that for creative and intellectual output, distractions and mental rest are necessary (Price, 2021). Allowing students time and space to be "lazy" can actually improve their learning.

Time & Control

When I was an undergraduate student, I worked as a campus tour guide and orientation leader for several years. Of all my several on-campus jobs throughout college, this was my favorite. The work was never boring: there were always new people, new conversations, new opportunities to share my knowledge and my genuine love for my small, public, liberal arts college. But there came one semester when my tour shift ended just as one of my classes started, and despite many efforts, neither could change. So every Wednesday morning, I was late to my 10:00 A.M. class. I could never smoothly end the full-campus tour and get to class on time, even though it only took about ten minutes for me to power-walk across the entire campus. The situation displeased both the admissions team and the professor. To my employer, the tours were always rushed—a fifty-minute tour was too fast. Campus tours were supposed to last *at least* an hour (and should ideally spill over an hour, apparently, an unspoken but nevertheless very real expectation of southern hospitality). To my professor, even with a formal letter from the Office

of Admissions, I was a nuisance, a disrespectful student strolling into class late and interrupting

lectures and discussions. I endured an entire semester of disdainful glares and snide remarks, and

the only reason I didn't lose points for tardiness was because I was desperate enough to ask the

Director of the Office of Admissions to write a letter on my behalf. I had an official-enough

"excuse" to keep my job from impacting my grade. Most students aren't so lucky: if it hadn't

been an on-campus job, my tardiness wouldn't have been excusable.

Students have all kinds of stories like mine, ones of unsympathetic teachers and of

struggles to meet the demands on their time. I remember getting locked out of a classroom in

middle school, and I remember myself as a student being judgmental about peers who seemed to

stroll into class late like they didn't care. The common conflation of punctuality and laziness

impacts more than education systems, it also impacts employment and professional

opportunities. People who show up late to class are deemed lazy; people who show up late to

work are deemed unreliable, untrustworthy, and unprofessional (by not contributing to the

capitalist work ethic in consistently normative ways). Time strictures are thus implemented in

academic settings to "prepare" students for the "real world," all while enculturating students who

will go on to enforce such ideologies in their professional lives. Within a given course there are

several time strictures: showing up on time, leaving on time, sitting patiently through several

class periods, finishing in-class work on time, getting across campus to the next class or job on

time, starting and submitting assignments on time, emailing the teacher with enough advance

notice to receive support, and now, with the increase in digital classrooms, logging on with

enough time for technological errors to resolve and updates to pass. My campus tour guide

anecdote demonstrates some of the difficulties many students have in balancing the demands of school and work, but it also showcases the ways in which constructions of time vary across contexts (and can directly conflict). Things like campus tours or lunch dates might not have strict timeframes, but in the classroom and especially in the submission of assignments, adhering to exacting time strictures is considered imperative for student success. Unforgiving attitudes of normative "timeliness" in educational settings ultimately aren't really about time itself, they are about control: schools controlling students, companies controlling employees. As part of their role and responsibility, teachers are charged with monitoring, scaffolding, allocating, and/or supplementing students' use of time. The issue, then, is examining what teachers are controlling and why, and what they can perhaps let go of without disservicing students.

One of my neurodivergent traits is time blindness, which is commonly described as the inability to accurately estimate, notice, or keep track of time. When paired with a trait attention scholarship calls "sluggish cognitive tempo" (Becker et al., 2022; Leikauf & Solanto, 2017), my relationship to time *really* doesn't match the norm. Non-normative time relationships are a common trait of autism and ADHD, and for me, it's more than just poor time management: it's sitting for six hours at my desk, writing and reading and hyperfocused and ignoring my body's needs; it's always being early or late to events, even with a friend or partner helping me stay accountable; it's getting in trouble at school as a child because I was happily daydreaming, or didn't complete a task in time, or didn't transition fast enough; it's consistently failing to prioritize or block out chunks of time in my day; it's the constant muscle-tensing anxiety about time passing because if I don't use additional tools to supplement my executive functioning (so I can focus on other things while still tracking the flow of time around me), I'm not as productive, and I get behind, and the anxiety spirals. One complex, consequential aspect of time blindness for me is having meetings or appointments ruin an entire day. If I have an appointment at 1 P.M., for example, my time-foggy brain has difficulty determining what I can feasibly accomplish before then—and not without precedent. If I have my spouse agree to remind me or set a timer/alarm on my computer, I can maybe complete a few tasks by then, with the relief of knowing my spouse or timer will remind me when it's time to get ready. But if I try to do something I enjoy or find interesting, like making an aesthetically pleasing presentation about reflective writing for transfer, I may get hyperfocused and lose track of time, and then suddenly it's 12:42, and maybe I still need to get dressed and pack my things (or, if I've remembered to do those things in advance, maybe it's putting on makeup or herding my cats out of the office or navigating worse-than-usual traffic), and then suddenly it's 12:55, and if I wasn't panicking before, I'm definitely panicking now. And then the tasks are interrupted and half-done, which halts whatever motivation I had, and who knows when that will come back.

When activities and events I enjoy wreak constant havoc in other aspects of my life, I begin enjoying those things less and less. I begin to fear *starting tasks at all*. I begin setting all my appointments for super early in the morning so I have less time to "waste" or fill with panic. There are all kinds of consequences for time-blind situations like these: some people may begin avoiding appointments entirely (or meetings, or fun events, or dates with friends); like me, some people will develop anxiety-related behaviors to ensure they aren't late; then, if they are late, especially chronically, there are even more consequences. They're considered lazy, disrespectful, unprofessional, and unmotivated. Sometimes they lose their job. Sometimes they don't have partners or friends to help them stay on track. Time blindness may seem trivial when it's reduced to "just" hyperfocusing or minor incidents like forgetting I've had tea steeping in the kitchen for over an hour. But in truth time blindness has compounding, far-reaching impacts on one's life. And while research shows most people aren't great at estimating how long a task will take to complete (Buehler et al., 1994, 2010; Wang & Chiou, 2022), my slow "processing speed" and other neurodivergent traits make time even weirder and more anxiety-inducing. For me, normative time either bleeds slow like a seaside fog or it races by like it's on the Talladega Superspeedway, laughing at me as it goes. Honestly, sometimes it doesn't exist at all.

My difficulties with time are in part mitigated by my generalized anxiety disorder. Until I developed depressive symptoms during and post-COVID, I was always the "eager" student who showed up early to class; I was the "good" student who took excessive amounts of notes and started my assignments as early as possible. These survival mechanisms are looked upon favorably by American academic and workplace cultures, so I was rarely externally punished for my neurodivergent traits. But there are an uncountable number of students who have a variety of different traits, coping mechanisms, and responses to the pressures to conform to normative time strictures. When teachers enforce grade-related penalties (or social penalties, such as locking students out of the classroom or mocking them), they're punishing not only neurodivergence but also everyone who has issues beyond their control that interrupt their schooling.

In disability culture, crip time is a concept that "refers to a flexible approach to normative time frames" (Price, 2011, p. 62). Like the word "queer," *cripple* has been revived and reshaped into a means of identification, action, community, and pride. According to Simi Linton (1998), "*Cripple, gimp,* and *freak* as used by the disability community have transgressive potential. They are personally and politically useful as a means to comment on oppression because they assert our right to name experience" (p. 177). Similarly, crip time can provide transgressive perspectives to normative relations to time, temporality, and timeliness. In tracing the connections between crip time and queer temporalities, Kafer argues crip time is not just a type of accommodation, it's a vital shift in mindset: "rather than bend the bodies and minds to meet the clock, crip time bends the clock to meet disabled bodies and minds" (2013, p. 27). Crip time isn't just affording students "extra" time (though many of us need it); crip time isn't just a joke about disabled people always running late (though we do sometimes joke about it). In her article "Six Ways to Look at Crip Time," Ellen Samuels (2017b) describes crip time as time travel, grief time, broken time, sick time, writing time, vampire time. I find so much value in these descriptions and their accompanying stories. Without crip time, we're syncopating—existing off schedule with the "regular world," breaking our minds and bodies to squeeze into normate shapes, grieving not only those we love(d) but that which we can never have, losing months to illnesses, perpetually realigning ourselves with narrow notions of linear time, mediating time and timeliness through various technologies.

In Tara Wood's (2017) article about crip time in writing classrooms, she reminds us that teachers must pay attention to how time is constructed in their classrooms: not just how much time is allotted per task, but also the structures around and implications of time allocations. How do I determine how much time is "enough" time for a specific task? Does timeliness factor into my assessment criteria (if so, *why*)? What are the consequences of tardiness, late work, or deadline extensions in my class? Do deadlines even exist in my class? Importantly: who benefits from normative expectations of time? Who doesn't? Wood writes, "The belief that student writers, given a set amount of time, have an equitable opportunity to perform in a way that suits their cognitive style and pace relies on an assumption of normativity" (2017, p. 269). To move away from such assumptions of student ability, cripping time in writing classrooms and writing assessment becomes a vital project.

The actual implementation of crip time in classrooms can be difficult for teachers—it often means letting go of control, and that can be scary for some. It also means radically trusting students, as I address in the forthcoming section of this chapter. When letting go of such control, some teachers fear that if they aren't carefully allocating students' time for them, complete with well-meaning penalties for noncompliance, students won't complete tasks and thus won't learn. In his blog article "Against Cop Shit," Jeffrey Moro (2020) argues for the abolition of "cop shit" in classrooms, which he defines as "any pedagogical technique or technology that presumes an adversarial relationship between students and teachers," with "militant tardy or absence policies" listed among such techniques. Cop shit operates within market logics, supports datafication of student information and performance, and offers order- and efficiency-based respites for teachers in a world full of seemingly scheming, unmotivated, chaotic students. The Laziness Lie further contributes to the allure of cop shit, making classrooms more about student management than co-construction of knowledge. Because learning is incredibly difficult to assess in an individual, let alone at scale, it's easiest to reduce learning to productivity (did you do all the things I asked), memorization (did you store the knowledge I imparted), and efficiency (did you not waste my time). Cop shit ensures compliance to such assessment loci. That's why it exists—enforcement. According to Moro (2020), cop shit is the antithesis of and actively prevents solidarity and community building between students and teachers. If teachers are too focused on managing their students' usage of time and their productivity, they can't build meaningful relationships or support their learning in accessible ways.

So when it comes to time, temporality, and timeliness, what are teachers controlling and why? And if grades exert a great deal of control over students, as we know they do, how are embedded normative timeframes contributing to that control? When normative time strictures are enforced, benevolently or otherwise, students whose bodyminds exist and learn outside of those strictures must learn to work around them or find ways to cope with the demands, many of which will require additional time and energy—or they will fail, slipping further into the toxic cycles of

avoidance, procrastination, shame, guilt, and fear.

Trust & Disclosure

adrienne maree brown (2017) reminds us to "Trust the People. (If you trust the people,

they become trustworthy)" (p. 42). Jesse Stommel (2017) says, "Start by trusting students."

These calls for trust always sound so intuitive. The instructors with whom I consult instinctively

assume they trust their students, but the moment we begin unpacking what that trust entails,

contingencies roll in. They recall memories of people cheating, lying, or "gaming the system,"

and those instances become evidence for control mechanisms. The blame and responsibility is

always placed on students; instructors never think to interrogate their own complicity in

structuring a distrustful learning environment. No one wants to hear that the way they design

materials or teach can facilitate or mitigate students' proximity to maladaptive learning

behaviors. In this section, I want to talk about radical trust: the kind of trustfulness that is

vulnerable and empathetic, that requires examining proximity to privilege and bigotry, and that

might be uncomfortable but is ultimately needed for justice-oriented classrooms.

During my first semester as an instructor of record, a funny thing happened: a student fell

asleep in class. The other students watched me warily, afraid of my reaction. I probably confused

them when I laughed, but I was genuinely more amused than offended. This was a true sleep, not

just a half-conscious nap situation, and it reminded me of undergrad and how I used to drag

myself and my friends to our early-morning classes. The other students and I collectively agreed

to leave the student alone. The exhausted student slept through our small group work and

discussions, and their friend woke them when the period ended. For me, this gesture was not just an extension of lenience or empathy, it was an intentional resistance of typical classroom protocols, which assume students who fall asleep in class are lazy, irresponsible, and inconsiderate of their peers' and teacher's time and energy. The Laziness Lie tells us such behavior is wasteful, too, in addition to disrespectful. But by letting the student rest without punishment, we prioritized their wellbeing. By resisting the inhumane demands on students' energy and time, our classroom welcomed non-normative ways of engaging in learning. Our composition program had a strict attendance policy at the time, and for that student on that particular day, being physically present in the classroom was truly their best effort. Who was I to punish them for it? If a student is tired enough to fall asleep (and *stay* asleep) in the midst of an in-person class, they quite obviously need the rest more than they do a lecture.

That student later disclosed that they had gone through extensive hazing that week; they apologized for falling asleep, and I assured them multiple times it wouldn't impact their grade. Other students in the class told me that my "lenience" that day reduced their fears about showing up late or being too tired to meaningfully contribute. Though I couldn't have articulated it at the time, this was an example of radical trust in practice: I didn't just *say* I trusted my students to be responsible for their own learning, I demonstrated that trust by resisting an opportunity to micromanage how they spent their time and energy. Rather than punishing the student, I trusted they would ask a friends for notes, access our class's shared lesson-plan notes, or ask me for details about what they missed. The student did all three.

An important locus of trust is student absences. As a new instructor of record, it didn't take long to develop strong feelings about students' relationship with disclosure. Almost immediately, I was horrified and exhausted by the amount of emails with self-deprecating apologies and requests for mercy via deadline extensions and the hopes of "excusing" absences/late work. Among colleagues, I also saw quite a lot of effort put into interrogating the validity of such excuses. It was a constantly evolving question: what counts as a "valid" excuse? As such, my students' pleas for humane pedagogical treatment were accompanied by disclosures of the deaths of loved ones, sudden temporary illnesses, flare-ups of disabilities or chronic illnesses, hospital visits, family emergencies, and other various medical, stressful, and/or traumatic events. I've heard a common joke in academic spaces about students having "multiple grandparents" pass away in one term, with the punchline being that students use the purported deaths of family members to cheat via requesting deadline extensions or some kind of attendance or grade policy leniency. And then COVID-19 happened, and suddenly teachers weren't joking about students losing family members anymore.

My sense of this phenomenon was always skewed, I guess: I was never that student (such is my email-related anxiety that I would've rather shown up with a 102 fever than email a professor). I also know that whenever one of my friends sent in "excuses" to their instructors to beg for extra time or some other type of humane treatment, they always had a reason, even if they didn't feel comfortable disclosing it to their instructor. My friends were either physically or mentally exhausted, especially my fellow student-athletes; or they were still recovering from an illness but should have been "better" by then; or they were devastated by a romantic breakup or another type of relationship ending; or they were dealing with familial troubles that didn't involve death but were still stressful or traumatic to manage, *especially* as a teenager. I had friends whose family members were arrested, or were dealing with drug or alcohol addiction, or were experiencing housing and food insecurity; I had my own minor family drama, but I also have chronic illnesses that mean my recovery time from "regular" illnesses, especially respiratory ones, is slower than average. When there's no trust between teacher and student, it's no wonder students lie about the realities of their messy lives.

Such disclosures are made necessary by a widespread mistrust of students as well as the habit of policing students' actions, behaviors, and use of time. Students don't succeed if they don't play by these rules. Mia Mingus (2011, 2017) calls this phenomenon "forced intimacy" (the opposite of "access intimacy") wherein disabled folks are required to share deeply personal details about their lives to attain the same level of access as those with normate bodyminds. "Disabled people are expected to 'strip down' and 'show all our cards' metaphorically in order to get the basic access we need in order to survive. We are the ones who must be vulnerable— whether we want to or not" (Mingus, 2017). The rampant skepticism of disability means disabled students are more likely to have to explain their personal circumstances (either with official documentation to campus disability services or to individual teachers, though often it's both). This forced intimacy Mingus describes gets shape-shifted into narratives of misfortune, tragedy, and/or inconvenience. Something to be overcome, or fix, or handle with resilience. Because of my own neurodivergent traits and the chronic stress/trauma of graduate school, learning to set boundaries around student disclosures was a matter of survival. Trusting my students was, for me, a matter of survival. Even before COVID-19, I implemented a blanket "I believe you! I don't need details, just tell me if you're ok and how I can help" communication policy, and later a blanket forty-eight hour deadline extension policy. Very quickly, there was more trust, more straightforward communication about students' needs and how I could support them, and more time spent focused on teaching and learning rather than policing.

Disclosure and trust have an interesting relationship: they aren't automatically concomitant, and they can either supplement or hinder each other. In disability studies, disclosure is understood as an ongoing process of revealing (or "proving," as Samuels discusses) one's disability or one's proximity to disability (Kerschbaum, 2019; Kerschbaum et al., 2017; Samuels, 2014). Disclosure can be many things, spoken or unspoken, visual or textual, and it has rhetorical power in some situations and doesn't in others (Samuels, 2017a). But in many cases, disclosure can be risky, unsafe, harmful. There are also many who, because of their appearance, may not have the option to consent to disclosure—their body/voice/assisting devices or personnel may disclose their non-normativity for them. Disclosure is an ongoing phenomena in writing classrooms not just for disability, but for queerness, poverty, documentation status, trauma, and so on. Application essays (especially "diversity" and needs-based funding applications) and literacy narratives are rife with such forced intimacies. Often, these essays are assigned without any critical attention to what teachers are actually asking students to do or *why* they're asking them to do it (Carello & Butler, 2014). For some of us, it can be painful to read (and give feedback on, and re-read, and worse, *evaluate for a grade*) these stories. When teachers think about how they design and assess such assignments, expectations of disclosure and consent should be just as transparent as other evaluative criteria. As Browning (2014) reminds us, composition teachers can do more to center disability justice frameworks in the structures of their pedagogy and grading practices (rather than just course content).

Simply put, trauma and oppression shouldn't be a currency exchanged for instructional clemency. Such conversations with students, if or when necessary, should be dialogues centered around mutual trust and respect. Students with disabilities, and all students, should not have to make such disclosures as a trade for deadline extensions or other accommodations; crip time and radical trust should be built into our pedagogical frameworks without the need for stories of trauma or oppression narratives. These issues with disclosure are often issues about trust: if there were mutual trust and respect, absences wouldn't be tracked as evidence of laziness and thusly punished, tardiness wouldn't be automatically penalized as indications of disrespect, and trauma narratives wouldn't need to be traded for teachers' benevolence.

It's not revolutionary to say there's a culture of mistrust in academia. As Moro (2020) explains, the adversarial relationship of students and teachers is not only antithetical to deep and meaningful learning, it's also symptomatic of a culture of surveillance, scarcity, and exertion of control. Turnitin and other companies profit quite literally from (and further perpetuate) teachers' mistrust in their students. Especially with the recent boom of AI writing technologies such as ChatGPT, there has been (and will likely continue to be) a surge of fear-mongering, doubt, and cynicism about student intentions and behavior around writing, plagiarism, and cheating. As AI writing tools improve and become more accessible and more intuitive, will teachers adapt, or will they continue using cop shit to monitor and punish students?

Developing a radically trustful classroom community is not an easy or natural endeavor. But, as I discuss in the forthcoming section, it's best to "fix systems, not people," especially when working within either a social justice or disability justice framework. Disability is socially constructed and reinforced through various norms of behavior and physicality—when we try to "fix" students, we are not only functioning within curative imaginaries (which reduce people to their disability, assume intervention to "fix" those people, and thus reinforce that disabilities are personal rather than structural problems) but also telling that student that they (and their disability) are the problem. Instead, we want flexibility, transparency, and, most importantly, we want structures that ask instead of assume.

Implementation

So far, I have put stories and scholarship to some of the ways neuronormativity is structured in writing classrooms. Through the Laziness Lie, students are enculturated to believe that their worth is intrinsically tied to their productivity and exhaustion, thus leading to behaviors like procrastination and avoidance; through time strictures and other measures of control, teachers penalize neurodivergence and maintain an adversarial relationship with their students, one that precludes avenues of more engaged learning; because of education's culture of mistrust, students are coerced into situations of forced intimacy, resulting in not only vicarious trauma or retraumatization of teachers but also the required use of students' trauma and oppression as currency exchanged for support. In these and many other ways, neuronormativity creates additional barriers for neurodivergent students, supports the disruption of meaningful teacher/student relationships, and prevents community building.

Though assessment is the focus of my intervention here, it must be reiterated that one cannot simply change one aspect of the classroom and suppose everything to be perfectly fixed or automatically equitable. All aspects of pedagogy interact and overlap in complex ways, and making an update to one aspect (which we chunk into discrete categories for ease of research and educator training) often requires updates to others. Adjusting our assessment tools and evaluative criteria often isn't enough. As Inoue (2015) suggests, for antiracist and social justice endeavors to be successful and sustainable, the entire assessment *ecology* must be attuned to those goals, not just the rubric or even the teacher or classroom itself.

That said, this section of this chapter is structured by and for practical recommendations. Disability studies and antiracist teacher/scholars are often loath to provide direct pedagogical suggestions for fear that readers will simply take these "quick tips" and not do any of the deeper personal reflective work or the broader classroom re-imagining that social justice pedagogies require. Of course, we cannot let complacency keep us in harmful racist, ableist, normative ruts. But because teachers of all experience levels, ages, and abilities sometimes need stepping stones toward justice-oriented models, I end this chapter with practical strategies for identifying, examining, and potentially redressing neuronormativity in writing classrooms.

I believe removing grading from classrooms will eventually be a requisite component of socially just pedagogies. Until then, here are a few ways to reconceive of, alter, or remove grading in your classroom. If I could go back in time and give a short list to myself at the beginning of my teacher journey, this is what I would give her:

- Separate feedback from grades. If you do nothing else, do this.

- You cannot design a rubric that will eliminate your unease with calculating grades based on racist and ableist criteria. As soon as you can, ditch grading altogether (Stommel, 2020, 2021b). It will make more sense to your writing-center-consultant brain.

- Explain your grading or ungrading (Kenyon, 2022) model thoroughly (multiple times and in multiple ways). Make *all* evaluative criteria transparent.

- Ask students for their input as often as possible and in multiple modalities/ways. Making design decisions without the key stakeholders involved is not in standing with design justice (Costanza-Chock, 2020a) and/or UX research/design principles.

- Assignment design and assessment design are two sides of the same coin, so continue thinking carefully about alignment between them. Good assignments can help facilitate better assessment of student learning and vice-versa.

- Ditch all cop shit (Moro, 2020) and punishment-related points.

- Be so much kinder to yourself.

This list is not, of course, exhaustive. In the rest of the chapter, I'll address each of these points in more depth, but I've organized the upcoming selection of strategies into three sections: Flexibility, Transparency, and Recursivity.

Flexibility

In their monograph *Building Access: Universal Design and the Politics of Disability*, Aimi Hamraie (2017) (they/them pronouns) troubles the notion of flexibility as "an instrument of standardization, normalization, and fit" (p. 41) and explains how modern conceptualizations of product design and "users" are derived from legacies of industrialism, capitalism, and eugenics. Hamraie historicizes their arguments with many examples from previous centuries, drawing connections between scientific and military discourse, productivity, rehabilitation, and definitions of citizenship. From this and other research, machines and other technologies were considered operationally inflexible, shifting the responsibility of adaptability on humans and their bodies (rather than the environment) (Hamraie, 2017). These industrial understandings of flexibility do still pervade institutions of education, assuming students fit into standardized structures, forcing assimilation, and blaming them when they don't or cannot adhere. Though human variation is more broadly accepted than it was in the past, and though many teachers do their best to celebrate difference and diversity, structurally shaping classrooms to be responsive to human variation can be difficult. Making it less difficult is one aim of this work.

For our purposes, an ethic of flexibility suggests that administrators and teachers create assessment *systems* that are flexible rather than *people* who are flexible. This ethic follows the "fix systems, not people" (Reed, 2018) premise, one I find crucial to all social justice endeavors. Flexibility requires that teachers' grading systems be negotiable and negotiated, that they're co-creating not just content knowledge but also evaluation practices. The goal is to design *with/alongside* rather than *for* our students (though there are of course limits to how much labor we should be asking students toward that end). In disability studies, the maxim goes, "Nothing about us without us" (Costanza-Chock, 2020b). The premise is simple enough: don't conduct research on any community, but especially "vulnerable" communities, without them. And not just with their approval, but with their direct involvement from the beginning. I think about this often with students: how often are students consulted in curriculum design, course design, or placement assessment design? Are they not the primary users/stakeholders? Rather than demanding our students to be resilient and resourceful to survive in academia, putting energy toward developing systems that do the bending for them—that is a step toward disability justice in education. As currie & Hubrig (2022) demonstrate, designing resilient course documents is a much-needed exercise in the disability justice paradigm of *care work* (Piepzna-Samarasinha, 2018). They write, "Resilient document design is born of a need to jettison the ableist violence of student resilience and the knowledge that it is our institutions that require further scrutiny, not our students" (currie & Hubrig, 2022, p. 144). They eschew one-size-fits-all pedagogies in favor of practices of crip community building (p. 132).

Practical Strategies

1. Implementation of crip time benefits all students (Wood, 2017). Here are a few ways to embrace crip time and begin examining your relationship to normative time strictures:

   a. Remove tardiness penalties and any shaming related to punctuality.

   b. Remove penalties related to lateness in any capacity, especially assignments.

       i.   Or, at the very least, provide a generous and transparent explication of what lateness entails. If there is negotiation, ensure it *never* hinges on submission of trauma narratives in exchange for leniency.

      ii.   If you're not comfortable with removing lateness penalties entirely, try implementing a 48-hour extension policy for all assignments.

c. Don't grade in-class work. Even completion grading (which can be useful in other contexts) assumes that all students will be comfortable with meeting or able to meet the criteria required in the short timeframe. Instead, ask yourself: What's important about completing this work in class? How does it benefit students? What's important about it being graded and/or timed? Does a summative assessment (a letter/number grade) of a student's in-class work facilitate learning?

d. Don't assume all students will be able to perform certain tasks in class within strict time frames, including activities like freewriting.

e. When possible, share lesson plans and class notes before and after class—some students learn best when they can be prepared for what the lesson will include, and some will want to access the lessons/notes days or weeks later.

f. Remove attendance policies or reduce their power in your grading system. Lack of physical presence doesn't mean lack of engagement, especially for students with chronic illnesses and disabilities.

2. Provide multiple points of entry for course content, assignment/project guidelines, and assessment criteria. This principle is essential to Universal design for Learning (UDL). According to CAST, the Center for Applied Technology (2018), UDL operates under the following three principles: Multiple Means of Engagement, Multiple Means of

Representation, and Multiple Means of Action & Expression. Some of the questions I ask myself *and* my students:

    a. Can my feedback, instructions, evaluation criteria, and course content be accessed in multiple (simple, actionable) ways?

    b. Are students learning through a variety of modalities, discourses, and times/spaces?

3. Incorporate maximum construct representation (Elliot, 2016). When designing evaluative criteria (I.E. rubric items), consider the broadest possible interpretation or version of that criterion—and then use that to make your assessment. We often delimit assessment *constructs* (the thing we're trying to evaluate for) by giving them narrow definitions rather than expansive ones. An example: an essay criteria requiring thesis statements to have no more or less than three points.

    a. Facilitating conversations with students about such things can be a fun and interesting way of learning, too: I.E. ask students to list all possible interpretations of "thesis statement" and see what they come up with!

    b. Similarly, if you find that a student's work doesn't fit neatly within the constraints of a particular assignment, don't penalize them for it. Rather, ask yourself is this constraint necessary to achieve the desired learning outcomes?

Transparency

Transparency for assessment means making your expectations and evaluation criteria as *accessible* and *actionable/usable* as possible. Moving beyond "clear" is crucial: students need instructions or criteria they can act on. As I discuss in the "Recursivity" section below, it helps to ask your students (anonymously, when possible) to describe the ways in which the criteria are not accessible/usable. You can then revise and continue improving on the usability of your instructions, assignment guides, assessment criteria, and more.

For me, transparency is also about denaturalizing systems of power. As a White, cisgender, temporarily able-bodied, neurotypical-passing woman, I have a great deal of privilege, and I can talk about systemic injustices with far fewer consequences than some of my colleagues. Once there is a sense of community, it can be useful to have students examine their proximities to privilege and power. When I ask students to do something like this, I model the exercise with an examination of my own privileges. (I try my best to never ask students to do something I would not do.) I openly discuss my White privilege, name it, and I disclose my neurodivergence and queerness. We discuss how privilege(s) can be salient in one context and nonexistent in another. For me, transparency about my privilege is a crucial part of co-creating assessment criteria and examining the prevalence of White language standards. And these, as we know from Schalk (2018) and others, are bound up tightly with ableist and neuronormative standards. It's always a gnarled bramble of relations to power and privilege, and detangling some of it alongside students is one way I go about creating community.

Practical Strategies

1. Explain your grading system on day one. You don't need a preset grading contract to spend time discussing your grading/evaluation methods and policies. Address how you will evaluate your students' writing, how you deal with "lateness," or, for example, how you plan to collaboratively create the evaluative criteria. Students may be confused, as most teachers don't take the time to explain how and why they grade the way they do.

But don't panic! Use this confusion as a learning moment to discuss why grading is considered so natural and neutral that no one talks about it.

2. One way to accomplish the previous strategy is to create a "grading" document separate from the syllabus that details how you will evaluate every assignment as well as your students' engagement with the course (attendance policies, revise and resubmit policies, peer review policies and expectations, etc.). My version of this document also notes that these policies are flexible and can be negotiated throughout the semester.

3. Transparency about communication expectations is equally vital. Do you answer emails on the weekends or after 9 P.M.? Do you expect students to provide specific reasons and/or documentation to excuse absences or late work? Do you expect students to instead provide the basics of what they plan to do or what need from you? Being explicit about your communication expectations can be a powerful way to set boundaries for yourself and provide usable instructions for students' communication.

Recursivity

Recursivity asks us to (re)iteratively reflect on and examine our assessment ecologies through analyses of power, purposes, places, people, processes, parts, and products, which are the seven interrelated elements constituting a writing assessment ecology (Inoue, 2015, p. 176). We must reflect on our writing program and pedagogies frequently, thoroughly, and with contemporaneous, anonymous student insight. This approach combines orientations from both writing assessment and UX methodologies. Feedback loops are essential to assessment theory (Huot, 2002), and concepts of reflexivity are grounded in feminist theory. bell hooks (1994) reminds us that, "The engaged voice must never be fixed and absolute but always changing, always evolving in dialogue with a world beyond itself" (p. 11). Social justice work, including teaching, does not end; we are constantly adapting to the world around us. In line with UX design methodologies, iteration on assessment designs with feedback from students is a crucial part of disability justice in the writing classroom.

Practical Strategies

1. Embrace (re)iterative and reflexive design by actively requesting students' feedback on the course, assignments, grading practices, and other relevant pedagogical practices.

2. There are many ways to invite student input. From passing out blank notecards in class, group conversations, one-on-one conferences, to in-depth digital surveys—choose what works best for you, your context, your students, your modality. One option is to provide short, informal, and anonymous surveys throughout the term. A sample of some informal questions I sometimes ask my classes at midterm:

    a. How do you feel about the overall workload of the course so far?

    b. How do you feel about the vibe of our classroom environment so far?

    c. How do you feel about the usefulness of the in-class activities so far? If you rate the usefulness as low, what would you prefer to do instead with our time together?

    d. Anything else you want me to know?

3. Implement what makes sense for the class. It won't always be possible to implement some of the feedback, but you can still *address* students' ideas and explain your rationales. Doing so demonstrates that you value their ideas and experiences, and it also gives students a means to:

a. Reflect on their learning, their time spent on the coursework, and the classroom environment;

b. Communicate those feelings or progress; and

c. Air grievances that might otherwise remain unexpressed and then curdle into resentment.

4. I have found this recursive aspect of my pedagogy to be one of the most interesting and most useful. Not only because I learn more about the students and my own teaching, but also because I add to my ever-expanding list of ways to be more accessible.

Conclusion

Ableist norms permeate academic spaces in so many quietly devastating ways: they stretch and sprawl silently beside me in class, taking up space; they follow me into my home, leaving traces even in the private corners of my life; they cling to our students' shoulders, burdening their movements, shaping their paths. They are challenging—not impossible—to shake off. I like to imagine myself taking out the trash and bringing my weekly accumulation of ableist violence with it: there are days when the task feels like a vital step toward self-compassion and community-focused care/access, and there are days when it feels infuriatingly Sisyphean. But denaturalizing areas of entrenched neuronormativity is only one of *many* ways to begin enacting crip community-building in our writing classrooms. It's also a particularly salient area of analysis for writing assessment, as so many of our grading habits rely on normative measures of time, labor, thinking, and writing.

As I discuss elsewhere in this dissertation, crip community-building is a practice of actively advocating for and/or generating localized collective care and access. With disability justice principles at the forefront, localization can take on new forms and create new opportunities for writing assessment. Addressing neuronormativity in writing classrooms can help teachers accomplish many things: identify and address biases; examine how those biases pervade our personal and professional discourse communities; examine how those biases inform our perceptions of ourselves and others, especially students; examine how those biases inform our teaching and especially our grading practices; examine how those biases are entrenched in and support our institutions and cultures at large. Like racial biases, disability biases are infused and interconnected with many other forms of oppression and discrimination, and disentangling them is the work of communities, not just individuals.

Through this work, I hope to offer teachers (and other academic administrators and practitioners) ways of addressing structures, not just individual practices or disability-specific solutions. We want—need—structures that do the bending and flexing for us. Let's create load-bearing structures rather than expecting load-bearing teachers and resilient students.

Chapter Five

CONCLUSION: REFLECTING ON
EXPERIMENTS OF CARE

I have been engaged with writing and reading for as long as I can remember. Prior to college, I had a dozen or so spiral bound notebooks filled with scribbled poetry and amalgams of creative nonfiction, fanfiction, and fantasy/sci-fi; as early as first grade, I was participating in every school-sponsored book-reading competition. Book fairs were my favorite event of the year. Writing and reading were spaces of comfort and catharsis, of escape and exploration, of practice and pursuit. Writing and reading gave my life direction when purpose was hard to come by; they were familiar ground in a world that was constantly shifting underfoot.

Yet for much of the schoolwork that came later, writing was a chore. I procrastinated on essay assignments and ignored injunctions to write in particular ways, but every small act of resistance was clobbered away through the ultimate mechanism of control in the classroom: grades. Circles instead of dots over my 'i's? Points off. Paragraph with four sentences instead of five? Huge mistake. Personal opinions where there ought to be relevant references to the text and connection to the three-pronged thesis? Letter grade down. It never ended, and it was always a moving target, year to year, teacher to teacher. For most of my life, I didn't understand why these things confused and frustrated me so badly. All I knew was that I needed to work harder, take better notes, make more flash cards, do better, *be* better.

College was both better and worse—I grew as a writer and reader, and I had more refined coping mechanisms, though I still didn't understand half the feedback I received. But at the tail end of my undergraduate career, I became a writing center consultant, and my perspective broadened. I learned how to evaluate without criticism, assess without assigning a grade, and facilitate a session via inquiry rather than dictation. I finally began learning to read rhetorically rather than critically. As an English major trained in literary criticism, learning how to facilitate growth in peer writing was an exciting challenge. No session was alike, even if the assignments were the same. With my official writing consultant title, my friends flocked to me like seagulls crying for chips, and I discerned a pattern. Everyone with whom I worked (both on and off the clock) had one thing in common: all they wanted was a better grade.

When I taught my own writing class for the first time, the professional expectations shifted—as an instructor of record, I was suddenly required to grade student writing. Despite my best efforts, I could not devise a way to do so without obliterating my sense of purpose, without damaging students' writing self-efficacy, or without making them hate writing more. Even with our communally constructed rubrics, mock-grading sessions with sample essays (to discuss genre conventions prior to dialogic rubric creation), class discussions of the slipperiness of grading writing, and entire weekends grading and crafting feedback with utmost care and conscious reminders of my own biases—no matter what I did, the grades spoke for themselves. No matter what pedagogical methods I tried or reassurances I gave, my students still focused on their grades, and they experienced them as value judgments about their abilities. When a grade is given, Brian Huot (2002) explains, "the person is the object of that articulation" (p. 62). But when we evaluate without a grade, score, or label, "the writing remains the object" of the evaluation. "Grading or testing," Huot goes on, "involves little or no learning or teaching" (2002, p. 62). I learned how, because of their social capital and high stakes, grades maintain primacy in students' affective experience of a writing course. I removed rubric grading where I felt I could and used our communal specifications-type rubrics, but I still spent my "grading weekends" having panic attacks on the floor of my apartment.

When I reached out to colleagues for guidance, I did so in small ways that, like usual, masked the extent of my anxiety: quick questions in the printer room, vague email requests for alternative rubric designs, and friendly chats over coffee in the break/printer rooms. In those conversations, I found spectrums of ambivalence and resignation (and sometimes ignorance). No one had the solutions I didn't know I wanted, and I couldn't articulate what I needed or why it mattered so much. But I remember it clearly: I experienced grading my students' writing as violence—I felt it in my chest, in my lungs, in my too-tense muscles. I felt the damage I was doing, and I hated it. And I had no idea why! I thought I just had a bad rubric.

I then came to the University of Arizona to begin my doctoral program, and I attended the required Writing Program General Meeting a few days before the beginning of the semester. If you ask anyone present in that library conference room on that kairotic day in August of 2018, you'll hear about Asao B. Inoue and his presentation on labor-based grading contracts. Depending on who you ask, you'll learn that we were told we are racist and that our grading practices are also racist. While partially true, Inoue's presentation was, like all his other work, incredibly holistic, well-researched, thoughtful, compassionate, and data-driven.

I'll never forget the program-wide resonance that followed in the days, weeks, months, and years to come. Inoue's presentation about labor-based contract grading described how systemic racism is naturalized not only in linguistic standards but *also* in assessment standards. That day, he encountered questions of resistance, and I listened, and I felt many things— terrified, excited, fragile (my and many others' White fragility went off the charts at being told, even compassionately, that we were enacting racial and systemic violence against our students without realizing it). But, mostly, I felt like I had been set free: there *were* alternatives to the irreconcilable, anxiety-producing tension between my pedagogical values and "standard" assessments. The frustration and discomfort I associated with grading were heightened by the lived realities of what I would later know as neurodivergence. Having panic attacks every time I went to grade student work; having moral/ethical crises every time I attempted to "justify" a rubric cell or grade number; having fellow instructors tell me "that's just the way it is"—it was all too much. And it wasn't what I had come back to school to do. Then, in one presentation, a leading scholar in the field basically said to me, "You know what? It doesn't have to be like this. In fact, it shouldn't be like this. Let's do better."

A few days later, I was introducing my students to a labor-based grading contract. With his permission, I used most of Inoue's system, and I had the support of Keith Harms, fellow assessment scholar as well as my preceptorship leader. At Inoue's recommendation, Keith and I also established a reading/discussion group to support other instructors attempting contract grading. The impeccable Eric House and Brad Jacobson, who both had been using alternative assessment models for years before Inoue's talk, facilitated a learning session and presentation about antiracist grading systems. That session challenged me to do better, to work harder to actively unlearn the White supremacy naturalized and neutralized in my White worldview, and to continue taking risks toward antiracism in the classroom. Much of what I know about alternative modes of writing assessment I learned from them and their mentorship.

Labor-based contract grading relieved the majority of my personal stress around grading writing, but not all of it. While I had several conversations with colleagues about Inoue's system and my frustrations with it, I found the most productive sessions were with my graduate cohort peers, especially those who were versed in disability studies scholarship and disability justice. Fellow doctoral students Jay McClintick and Griffin X. Zimmerman had insightful critiques, and their research interests were an entry point into disability studies, a field I didn't even know existed. Griffin and I then collaborated on an article about neurodivergence and labor-based contract grading, and my research paths solidified from there. The frustrations I felt when transitioning from tutoring to teaching invoke tensions about grading that are not new (Elbow, 1994; Tchudi & NCTE, 1997; Huot, 2002; Moreno-Lopez, 2005; Kohn, 2012). Portfolio assessment, course contracts, and many other solutions have been proposed to address some of these concerns, including Inoue's labor-based contract grading model (2019). The current trend toward ungrading, or the removal of grades from the classroom completely, recognizes the harm grading causes and seeks alternatives (Blum, 2020). Moving toward these aims is a vital project of anyone seeking a more equitable classroom for their students.

This dissertation bridges justice-oriented principles between writing assessment and placement, disability studies, and user experience (UX) research/design methodologies in technical and professional communication (TPC). Little work has been done to incorporate disability justice in writing assessment scholarship, and too few assessment and placement systems are created in concert with substantive student input. Instead, we see assessment technologies and placement processes being imposed upon students rather than designed with them, and we see neuronormative models of grading writing that (de)limit opportunities for self-assessment. From a decolonial participatory design perspective (Agboka, 2013; Agboka 2014), to deny students opportunities to participate in the creation of systems that impact their enrollment, retention, and success (Adams et al., 2009; Inoue, 2009a; Valentine et al., 2017) is to further enact systemic oppression and harm (Lederman & Warwick, 2018). Additionally, writing studies lacks models addressing neurodiversity in writing assessment (Carillo, 2021; Kryger & Zimmerman, 2020). This dissertation addresses this need.

Chapter 2 utilizes the neurodiversity paradigm and the concept of neuronormativity to frame an analysis of three equity-oriented models of validity. This chapter offers a critical overview of the history of validity in writing assessment and its connections to the field of educational measurement and psychometrics. I also provide discussions of how validity comes from a history of positivism that no longer fits the current paradigms of writing studies or disability justice. I then examine three orientations to validity (consequential validity, racial validity, and fairness in validity), which I follow with an offering for considering validity through a disability justice lens and ways to move forward.

Chapter 3 positions directed self-placement (DSP) as a type of technical and professional communication (TPC) and argues that students ought to be considered "users" of these technical systems. Positioning students-as-users and DSP-as-TPC expands the realm of possibility for research and scholarship on student self-placement models and the usefulness of usability studies, participatory design, and user experience (UX) methodologies. The chapter provides an overview of the history of DSP and how it has become the standard for equitable writing placement. I then offer examples and stories of how we have implemented UX research/design in our DSP system here at our institution, demonstrating the potential variety and feasibility of UX research, usability, and participatory design methodologies for writing programs.

Chapter 4 returns to the neurodiversity paradigm and the overwhelming prevalence of neuronormativity in writing classrooms. After providing some key definitions and situating them within personal experiences, this chapter addresses harmful neuronormative assumptions and structures in writing classrooms, separated into three categories: Laziness & Procrastination, Time & Control, and Trust & Disclosure. Each of these topics resonates with my personal experiences as a student, teacher, and administrator, and I offer narrative pathways through this chapter that I hope are more widely accessible than the previous two chapters. I end this chapter with an Implementation section, which offers many practical suggestions for teachers to consider for moving toward a more anti-ableist classroom.

Future Research

The future of writing assessment will continue this journey toward equity, liberation, and social justice. More specifically, it will facilitate learning without the violence of grades or the limitations of normative assessments. As student populations become increasingly diverse, teachers of all ranks and disciplines will need new ways to support students whose experiences, talents, and dreams don't align with White, cishetero, able-bodied, middle-class, Christian norms. The institutions, programs, and departments who support these teachers and students must grapple with these changes too, and they must support their educations in doing so. Writing assessment happens across so many sites, so the avenues for future research seem endless, and my ADHD brain buzzes excitedly with the plethora of possibilities. But for the purposes of this project, I will provide a few of the most salient avenues for future study, which I consider to be ungrading, self-assessment, and large-scale assessment.

For classroom writing assessment, ungrading is growing in popularity as an alternative to traditional grading, grading contracts, specifications grading, and portfolio grading. Some call it "going gradeless," while others call it "de-grading," but the premise is all the same: the removal of all grading to the extent possible (with the understanding that many schools still require a final course grade) (see Blum, 2020). In removing grades from writing classrooms, students are asked to practice assessing their own work, as many gradeless classrooms rely on self-assessment and reflection as the alternative (in addition to ongoing formative feedback from instructors). An ungrading classroom can take many shapes and may use a combination of alternatives to traditional rubrics or grading methods. But at its core, ungrading requires many of the principles or ideas I have addressed in this dissertation, including but not limited to:

- Fundamentally trusting students;

- Relinquishing control, especially attachments to perceived "accuracy" or "fairness"; and

- Prioritizing student needs and humanity over institutional demands.

These are just three of potentially many aspects of a justice-oriented and gradeless classroom, and I see ungrading as being particularly responsive to the goals of crip community building and flexibility as access. When grades are removed and student learning is prioritized (rather than scores or other measurements of the learning), there's more room to be flexible. For example, when grades are removed and reflective self-evaluations are used, the evaluation of learning scales to the individual students and their needs, rather than trying to fit students' wildly different journeys into fixed letter or numerical grade systems. In this case, teachers thus relinquish their expectations of perceived objectivity and accuracy of their assessments in exchange for the flexibility of dialogic and emergent student learning goals, regressions (a natural part of the learning process; see Beaufort, 2007 for a discussion of negative transfer), and external factors of life that impact students' learning throughout their educational careers.

As mentioned above, I also see self-assessment as an important area of study in the future of writing assessment. As Huot (2002) notes, assessment is already a part of languaging (whether we attribute grades to it or not, we are always assessing our language use), and to write well, one must be able to assess that work. To dismiss that aspect of the writing process is to disservice our students. Self-assessment also aligns well with ungrading and many other socially just classroom assessment systems (Stommel, 2017; Blum, 2020). In the field of writing studies, we value the role and usefulness of reflection, particularly in that it supports aspects of metacognition and transfer (Beaufort, 2007; Taczak & Robertson, 2016). Finally, through portfolios, teachers are already facilitating this kind of (meta)cognitive reflection work, and enriching our understanding of how portfolios and self-assessment interact could benefit the development of more robust alternative assessment systems. But self-evaluation is best paired with peer review and other forms of teacher, community, and/or interpersonal interactions so students don't assume writing and assessment happen only in isolation. Such a multiplicity of feedback modes, combined with other efforts at challenging racist and ableist normativities in writing and thinking, may also help mitigate (or, at the very least, challenge) any internalized oppression or shame present in the self-assessment. For these reasons, self-assessment is an area ripe for further research in writing classrooms, particularly regarding how it connects to low-stakes writing, transfer, metacognition, portfolios, and equitable writing assessment.

Finally, doing any justice-oriented writing assessment work at scale—such as at the program, department, or institution level—is incredibly challenging. Though writing program and writing center administrators have been tending to this topic for some time (Adler-Kassner & O'Neill, 2010; Schendel & Macauley, 2012; White et al., 2015), there's still much to be learned from disability theory and activism in terms of coalitional leadership, justice-forward goals and design, and community building across diverse contexts. Directors of writing/learning centers, Writing Across the Curriculum (WAC) programs, and writing programs are often responsible for facilitating large-scale assessments, a recursive process that involves staff members, students, and other administrators across campus. The stakes are high, with funding, jobs, and program continuance at risk, and often the assessment process is fraught with concerns of time, labor, competing interests, and conflicting stakeholders. There are no simple answers to projects at such a scale, and there must be some level of advocating for what is needed to complete the assessment successfully and equitably. Whether that is additional time or additional funding to compensate participants/those doing the labor, building coalitions of dedicated people around mutual goals can help disperse labor. There absolutely should be more research on large-scale assessments and justice-oriented methodologies.

These and other avenues demonstrate the ways in which writing assessment and pedagogy has room to grow to better support an increasingly diverse and increasingly overburdened student population. Putting the labor of classroom justice methodologies solely on the shoulders of individual teachers is a recipe for burn out, chronic stress, and teachers leaving for other work. Putting effort into creating sustainable, humane, and highly flexible structures will, ideally, absorb rather than create more labor for everyone. But sometimes that means undoing and/or redoing what's been in place for extended periods of time, and that's difficult work in its own right. These experiments of care, as currie and Hubrig (2022) call them, are offered in the spirit of seeking this goal: leaving no bodymind behind.